TRADITIONAL KNOWLEDGE OF HOUSEHOLD PRODUCTS

TRADITIONAL KNOWLEDGE OF HOUSEHOLD PRODUCTS

by

Dr. Ashis Kumar Ghosh
M.Sc., M.Ed., Ph.D.,
Diploma in Naturopathy
H.M., Habibpur Saraswati Vidyamandir, Midnapore,
Paschim Medinipur-721101 (West Bengal)

2011
DAYA PUBLISHING HOUSE®
Delhi - 110 035

ISBN 81-7035-686-5
ISBN 978-81-7035-686-8

Published by : **Daya Publishing House**
1123/74, Deva Ram Park
Tri Nagar, Delhi - 110 035
Phone: 27383999
Fax: (011) 23260116
e-mail : dayabooks@vsnl.com
website : www.dayabooks.com

Showroom : 4760-61/23, Ansari Road, Darya Ganj,
New Delhi - 110 002
Phone: 23245578, 23244987

Laser Typesetting : **Twinkle Graphics**
Delhi - 110 088

Printed at : **Chawla Offset Printers**
Delhi - 110 052

PRINTED IN INDIA

Dedication

The author dedicates this work to the memory of
late Abinash Chandra Ghosh
(great grandfather, former headmaster during
1906–1914 of Rajagram
S.B. Raha Institution, P.O. Rahagram,
Bankura which is previously known as
Rajagram A.S. School) and to late
grandfather Bhutnath Ghosh, starter of
Calcutta Tram Company and
to my Parents.

Dr. K.P. Biswas
M.Sc., Ph.D., D.F.Sc. (Bom.)
F.Z.S. (Cal.), E.F. (W. Germany)
Former Joint Director of Fisheries, Govt. of Orissa
Director of Fisheries A&N., Admn., Govt. of India.
Visiting Professor :
W.B. University of Animal & Fisheries Science

Foreword

Sustainable ecofriendly management, the age old practices of the orient, which was suppressed by the influence of western method of practices is now gaining popularity among the western countries itself. Still today, traditional knowledges continue to be an important source for ecological development throughout the world. People in general are now prefer to use natural products. In this perspective, unwritten and undocated traditional practices has tremendous potentialities.

Practically there is no book on this subject hence Dr. Ashis Ghosh's book on "TRADITIONAL KNOWLEDGE OF HOUSEHOLD PRODUCTS" I presume, will help in guiding those methods of much needed measure for mankind.

Dr. K.P. Biswas
Former Joint Director of Fisheries,
Govt. of India.

Acknowledgements

I am privileged to record my gratitude to Prof. Sabyasachi Chatterjee of Kalantar Patrika, Joydev De (Asstt. Director), Swaswati Sen (Director of WWF), Jayanta Singha (Bajaj Alianz), Dr. Shyamapada Pal, Prabodh Panda (M.P.) for their keen interest in this work. My sincere thank is also due to my colleagues and M.C. members of Saraswati Vidyamandir for their encouragement. In the preparation of this book I have received valuable suggestions from the following persons : Dr. Madhup De. (A.D. I/S, Paschim Medinipur), Subrata Maity (A.I/S), Dr. Subhasis C. Patra, Dr. Debal Deb., Debdulal Bhattacharya, Sanchita Sau, Debu Das, Chanchal Mashanta (H.M.), Krishna De Pradhan (A.I/S), Rubi Chakraborty (A.I/S), Gopenath Das, Father Joy C.D. Souza (H.M.).

Author wants to express his thanks to Sarathi Maity (A.I/S), Priyanka Ghosh, Priyabrata Ghosh, Biplab Ghosh and Soma Ghosh for the patience shown by them during the preparation of the manuscript. Thank is also due to all the staff of D.I. office for their encouragement.

Dr. Ashis Kumar Ghosh

Preface

Due to industrialization alongwith mechanical life dealing a rapid change in human life leaves a snag in the establishment of harmony with nature as well as on the ecosystem and thereby damage ecosystem due to wide usage of chemical pesticides, fertilizers, plastic, synthetic drug etc. As a rest the long term detrimental effects, were exhibited. At present it has been indispensable to look for alternative sustainable ecofriendly approaches and the present book is an positive effort to mobilize in right direction. In this book knowledge is applied to saving nature and as a part of that to using resources more efficiently in order that all the creatures including man can live decent lives without wiping out the resource base. To do this and even to understand deeply the actual uses of traditional knowledge has been focused. Besides the book provides insight into some, aspect of the past, method for the present and guideline for future. It should be very helpful for the ecologists. Traditional Knowledge is not separate companion of life. The development of sustainable management starts from tapping the indigenous wisdom after establishing rapport with the indigenous people.

The research work incorporated in the book has been carried out by thorough survey in the selected places of West Bengal and its adjoining areas. Some of the works has already been published in reputed journals of India and Abroad. I do hope the book shall serve as a useful tool to the research scholars, teachers, students, doctors and laboratories alike.

No inconsistencies might have crept in.

Doljatra **Dr. A.K. Ghosh**

CONTENTS

1

Introduction

I have spent a large part of my life studying the indigenous knowledge and its application for living beings to maintain the ecological balance. I have realised that despite all the advancements in science, the scope for rejuvenating traditional knowledge systems remains ahead. Though within our national policy, the emphasis on the potential of indigenous knowledge has not been so high. The information available from our own experience has been put forward primarily to encourage the emerging naturalists. The process of converting an idea into prototype, product and enterprise is very critical. Sometimes indigenous knowledge provides an alternative ecofriendly model for rural development, employment generation and poverty alleviation based on augmenting innovation by small farmers, potters, sweet-makers, artisans, folkmen etc.

Foods and the eating practices of people are very much integrated into the overall heritage of the culture. Traditional food systems have the potential to enhance the quality of life. The need is to document and preserve traditional food systems. Further researches are needed for understanding the food diversity of Bengal and for proper utilization of indigenous knowledge in promoting the use of traditional foods. Keeping this in view, a maiden effort has been made in this book. It provides a voice to economically poor but knowledge rich communities and individuals.

Naturalists prefer not to use chemical pesticides and fertilizers, synthetic drugs, plastic, fibres etc., but preferring 'natural' remedies and resources. So extensive effort has been made in this context. Among the many facets of physiochemical events, nothing is more interesting than the study of senescence as it not only tells us the mystery of death of an organism but also gives an understanding about the different aspects of correlative plant behaviour which shows wide biological diversity, has been studied.

Besides continuity of global warming due to emission of Green House Gases has become a major environmental issue of the present day. The temperature is gradually raising, the glaciers are pouring their fresh water load into the ocean and the mankind is helplessly waiting for the last hours to face the disruption of food web. Considering all, the present book is an extensive effort to cater the basic knowledge for sustainable development. Environmental courses have been part of formal education since the 1960s, but this has clearly not been sufficient. The aim of this publication is to highlight the role of education in achieving a sustainable society.

Things to Remember

We are now facing enormous challenges. The number as well as population size of the planet's 1, 313 species of wild vertebrates (reptiles, birds, mammals etc.) is diminishing, the amount of man made chemical substances is increasing and as a result the climate is changing. As many as 37 football ground of tropical rainforest disappear in every minute, 45000 dams have a negative impact on nature, more than 1 billion people do not have access to drinking water.... and the list is endless. If we continue with the same unsustainable consumption and production pattern, by 2050 we would need 2 planets.

Humanity's ecological footprint is increasing. Our ecological footprint is too big. Since 1980s we consume the world's natural resources at a rate that is 25% faster than nature's capacity to create new ones. Today we produce more waste than nature can deal with, which means that we outstrip nature's capacity to create new resources.

Everyday we impart our environment in different ways, for *e.g.*, when we buy food, drive cars or heat our homes. We affect our surroundings and leave a so called ecological foot-print.

The average North American ecological footprint is 9.4

The average European ecological footprint is 4.8

The average Asian ecological footprint is 1.3

The average African ecological footprint is 1.1

The average World ecological footprint is 1.8
hectares per person.

How One Can Reduce His Ecological Footprint

A lot of things can be done through reducing product consumption, reducing car travel, eating more vegetarian food, changing to sustainable energy systems, buying eco-labelled products, supporting environmental organisations, buying secondhand clothes etc.

Western lifestyle puts a tremendous burden on the environment. Except a few country lifestyle the world's present development is unsustainable. If we are successfully address the world's problems and possibilities we need to equip ourselves to act for a more sustainable future and to live in harmony with nature. Sustainable development does not only mean ecological sustainability but also includes social and economic dimensions. Sustainable development meets the needs of the present without compromising the ability of future generations to meet their own needs. Besides sustainable development can be regarded as a journey *i.e.* an ongoing process within an ecological framework. The long-term objective is to have a good life as possible without hampering other living beings, nature and society in both time and space. An economy that is socially unjust or that does not correspond to the ecological framework is not sustainable. In a nutshell, acting sustainably makes economic sense. An economic development means economic benefits for society as a whole and that does not pose a threat to artificial and natural capital.

There are so many definitions, and steps of sustainable development. Such as (*a*) care for ourselves, (*b*) care for others (*c*) care for planet, (*d*) care for offsprings and so on. In a global perspective every person seems tiny. But lots of tiny people can make an incredible difference.

Bees and wasps know that the hexagon is the strongest and most flexible shape. They are genetically programmed to construct one cell after another in hexagonal patterns in order to provide the best possible conditions for future generations. In every moment through informal education we learned so more from the natural events. Future generations must be able to cope with the changes through incorporation as education for sustainable development. As learning is an ongoing process and life long so acquiring knowledge might be a demanding and tedious process but it is nevertheless easy to carry–it fits nicely into the body and is personal. Keeping in view "Every sunrise ought to be seen as a new opportunity, every day as a new challenge to secure our planet and its life forms for future generations. Despite all the alarms and investments in intensive environmental work our Earth is still deteriorating.

"The earth has enough for man's need but not for man's greed."
Mahatma Gandhi

"It would be good to live without spoiling things for others."
Wolfgang Brunner

Organic Farming for Sustainable Management

Diversity of plant life is the key factor on organic farms. Besides diversity is essential for soil health. Generally the groundcover provides shade on sunny days, while leaf litter cools the surface of the soil. High humidity under the canopy of nature long-life trees reduces evaporation and minimizes the need for irrigation. The droping leaves of trees act as a water meter to indicate falling moisture levels.

By ruining the natural soil fertility we actually create expensive artificial needs. So, now a days many farmers who are turning back on the increasingly industrialised means of agricultural production that needs costly input and taken to organic farming. In this way entire web of life must be protected and nurtured. While organic farming is supposed to be eco-friendly, someone have expressed fears over its possible adverse ecological effects. "We cannot feed 6 billion people with organic farming; if we tried to do so we will level most of our forests" said Norman E. Borlaug, father of the Green Revolution and Nobel Laureate. John Emslay a British Chemist said that the human race will face this century is not global warming but a global conversion to organic farming which would result in the perishing of over 2 billion people. Though India has enough food to feed her population of 1 billion plus, yet hunger and food insecurity at household level have increased. Now farmers unable to pay back debts incurred by the purchase of seeds, pesticides, chemical fertilizers and equipments kill themselves. Generally majority of them have committed suicide because they are steeped in debt, from loans taken to sow improved seeds or use better fertilizer or pesticide, or most likely a combination of all the three.

So, organic farming can prove profitable if we return to traditional practices. Now it is most necessary to monitor the health of the soil and thereby increased the beneficial microbial activity. Just I can say "If you save the soil, you save the nutrient. Since many of the developed and developing countries are land-starved, they should immediately switch over to organic farming. The arguments arises that organic farming requires more land. Holds good only for cash crops according to FAO.

In organic farming legumes are grown for N_2-fixing, and inter-cropping, crop-rotation, compositing, vermiculture, and so on, are practised to retain moisture and nutrients. Food productions of today are heavily subsidised. Organic food, since it does not receive any of these subsidies, in comparison, comes across as being found expensive. If the same subsidies are given like that of non-organically grown foods, and is perhaps likely to be cheaper in view of its superior yield. As a consequence widespread adoption of organic farming is unlikely to materially impact the availability of food. To begin with the practice of organic farming should be for low volume high value crops like medicinal plants, fruits, vegetables and spices. As a sustainable means of agricultural production and to promote health instead of spreading toxins through chemical fertilizers and pesticides Indian farmers of remote villages are still engaged with the traditional practice of organic farming.

Green Chemistry a Healthy Way

Several environmental laws have been passed to protect the environment by controlling our exposure to hazardous substance. Instead of limiting risk by controlling our exposure to hazardous chemicals green chemistry attempts to reduce and preferentially eliminate the hazard thus negating the necessity to control exposure. If we do not use or produce hazardous substances then the risk is nil. The fundamental idea of green chemistry is that the designer of a chemical is responsible for considering what will happen to the world after the agent is put in place. Green chemistry has gained a strong footprint in both industry and academia. The design of environmentally gracious products and processes are guided by 12 fundamental approaches of green chemistry to achieve the goals. Many of them are mentioned below :

1. **Prevention :** It is better to prevent waste than to treat the waste after it is exposed.
2. Less Hazardous Chemical Synthesis that possess mild or no toxicity to human health and the environment.
3. Designing eco-friendly chemicals.
4. Designing safer solvents and Auxiliaries (separation agent etc.).
5. Use of renewable feedstocks rather than developing.
6. Reduce unnecessary derivatives whenever possible.
7. Design for energy efficiency *i.e.* energy requirement should be minimized.
8. Design for degradation of the chemical products as a result no harmful end products can persist in the environment.

9. Inherently safer chemistry for accident prevention to minimize the releases, fires and explosions.

As green chemistry represents our sustainable future so the coming generation of scientists and research scholars need to be trained for eco-friendly techniques. Besides important steps to be taken for green chemistry within the school and college curriculum through the following approaches :

(*a*) Incentives to students for working on the projects of green chemistry.

(*b*) Organizing workshops and training courses.

(*c*) Introduction of the basic concepts of chemical toxicology and the basis of hazards.

(*d*) Incorporation of green chemistry topics within the professional examinations etc.

The future challenge for chemists as well as for the scientists is to develop products, processes etc., in a sustainable way to improve quality of life of living beings in accordance with the ecological rules.

2

Sustainable Folk Food

2.1 Amusing Medicinal Sweetmeats of Bengal

Abstract

Bengal is one of chief sweetmeat makers of India where so many varieties of sweetmeats are available since seventeenth century as the Bengalees are sweetmeat lovers. In addition to the major medicinal plants are also available in this state. The famous "Motichur" sweet of Bengal is confined only in historical Bishnupur.

The Global consumption of herbs as medicine, food, additive etc. is increasing rapidly. One of such area of high commercial potential medium is sweetmeat. Numerous compounds of plant origin are reported to have different degrees of curative property. In the light of limitations of currently marketed deleterious sweetmeat as well as drastic reduction of high calorific sugarmeat consumption especially in developed countries, an area of low calorific, less sweetener is gaining commercial significance. For commercialization of herbal sweetmeats in food industry, it needs to undergo rigorous evaluation. The present article is a compilation of information on medicinal intense natural sweetmeats derived from various plant parts, and this study list the herbal sweetmeats and their medicinal uses for further exploration.

Keywords : *Sweetmeat, Biosweet, Diabetic, Motichur.*

Introduction

Since ancient times so many efforts have taken to improving

food palatability. However, changing life style and sugar related health problems like obesity, dental caries and unsuitability of sugars for diabetic patients, replacement of traditional high calorific sugarmeat by low calorific intense sweetmeat has become essential. So, search for alternative as nutritive intense sweetmeats derived from plant (Douglas and Djendoel 2002). These natural ideal sweetmeats should be of low calorific value, able to mask the taste at lower concentration, full of antioxidant, energy potential and it should be free from health hazards, very suitable for long-term use, remain stable at wide range of temperature and pH.

Approaches similar to the ethnomedicine discovery programme exploring new sweetmeats from plants is very interesting. However, some specific taste perception are added advantage. Ethnomedicinal information derived from early literature can be a rational way in exploring new sweetmeats. Interview with employees of Sri Krishna sweets (Asok Nagar, 24 Parganas) and Hindusthan sweets (Jadavpur, Kolkata) Industry give an idea about herbal sweetmeats. However, the information from the above sources is not sole and still so many plants may remain unexplored in Bengal. Though several herbal sweetmeats of low calorific value have recently evolved as so many health hazards present in traditional sweetmeats (Inglett 1976, Sardesai and Waldshan 1991). Here promising plant parts with beneficial property is used. Safety assessment can be judged from threshold sensory method using healthy volunteers. Any compound with proven efficacy and safety can directly be used as sweetmeat. By chemical modification of natural plant parts or derivatives with improved potency, stability and reduced health hazards can also be prepared. Further, by using natural herbs new sweetmeats can be discovered.

Modern people prefer healthy bio-sweets which are mild sweety as body is the product of good habits alongwith nutritious food and drink. An attempt has been made to ventured in Indian sweetmeat industry, into arranging a negotiation between herbs and some indigenous items of sweets.

Materials and Methods

Sweetmeats made by machine from different freshly collected parts of herbs in "semi-automatic canning plant" for packing ladoos, rosogollas, gulabjam, sandesh, motichur etc. The grinding of ingredients is done by the semi-automatic grinding machine. The chhana balls are, cooked in herbal sweetener syrup. The famous sweet 'Motichur' of Bishnupur (Bankura) discovered by Mallaraj during seventeenth century at the period of second Raghunath Singhadeb made from fruits of piyal (*Buchanania lanzan*).

Conclusion

The demand of low calorific sweetmeat is gaining gradually not only because of sugar related health hazards but also due to rising number of diabetic patients especially in Bengal. Thus the extensive research work are necessary for the search of new sweetmeats from various biodiversified parts of Bengal. To ensure fruitful result anticipation is required from phytochemist and exhibition of herbal sweetmeats categorically linked for diseases to get benefit of this dual roles.

Table 1

Name of Herbs	*Parts Used*	*Botanical Name*	*Type of Sweet*	*Herbal Remedy of Biosweet*
Kulekhara	Leaf	*Hygrophila spinosa* (Acanthaceae)	Curd, Rosogolla	Excessive bleeding, anaemia, kidney and gall stone, jaundice, insomnia, herpes.
Arjun	Bark	*Terminalia arrjuna* W and A (Combretaceae)	Rosogolla, Golabjam	Reduced blood sugar, blood pressure, white discharge, spermatorrhoea, blood dysentery, cardiac asthma, anaemia, cirrohsis of liver, heart stimulant.
Brahmi	Leaf	*Bacopsa monnieri* (Scrophulariaceae)	Curd, Rosogolla	Epilepsy, ulcers, dyspepsia, flatulence, constipation, asthma, sterility, general debility, intellect promoter.
Carrot	Root	*Daucus carota* (Umbelliferae)	Ladoo	Dyspepsia, colic pain, cardiac, debility, cough, asthma, bronchitis, diabetes, jaundice, diuretic, night blindness (boiled juice of carrot root mixed in boiled milk in 1 : 1 ratio to make nutritious curd and ice cream).
Tulsi	Leaf	*Ocimum sanctum* L (Lamiaceae)	Curd, Rosogolla	Cough and cold, pox and measles.
Susni	Leaf	*Marsilea minuta* L (Marsileaceae)	Rosogolla	Insomnia, epilepsy, asthma, loss of memory, high blood pressure.
Soybean	Seeds	*Glycine max* L. (Fabaceae)	Curd, Rosogolla	Reduces uric acid, cholesterol, blood pressure, sodium levels.

(Contd...)

Name of Herbs	*Parts Used*	*Botanical Name*	*Type of Sweet*	*Herbal Remedy of Biosweet*
Pudina	Leaf	*Mentha viridis* L (Lamiaceae)	Beverage, Rosogolla	Indigestion, gastric ulcer, dyspepsia.
Water melon	Fruit	*Citrullus vulgaris* (Cucurbitaceae)	Beverage, Rasogolla	Diarrhoea, dysentery, sunstroke.
Water chestnut (Bulls' head)	Fruit	*Trapa bispinosus* L (Hydrocaryaceae)	Singharah	Low caloric diabetic food used in singarha and is an alternative of wheat.
Date palm	Fruit	*Phoenix dactylifera* L (Arecaceae)	Rosogolla	Antisenescence, antiabortic, spermatorrhoea.
Black Berry	Fruit	*Syzygium cumini* L (Myrtaceae)	Ladoo	Antidiabetic and antiglycemic.
Piyal	Fruit	*Buchanania lanzan* (Anacardiaceae)	Motichur	Cold, cough.
Papaw	Fruit	*Carica papaya* (Caricaceae)	Ladoo	Dispepsia.
Beet	Root	*Beta vulgaris* (Cruciferae)	Ladoo, sandesh	Dispepsia.

2.2 Traditional Sweetmeats and Beverages of West Bengal

Abstract

Indigenous technical knowledge (ITK) on the various sweetmeats and beverages has been communicated which are still existing. Sweetmakers normally process the sweetmeats for income generating and nutrient supplementation. The study describes the traditional sweetmeats of indigenous people of W. Bengal and documented them for the welfare of tourists and for future generation before abolishing. The sweetmeats reflect the socio-cultural, ecological and spiritual life style of Bengalees. Besides W. Bengal is rich in beverages and sweetmeat diversity those play an important role in the life of Bengalees.

Keywords : *Indigenous knowledge, Motichur, Mallaraj, Haria.*

Introduction

Sweetmeats and beverages are the necessary commodity both for life sustenance and cultural status. The social facets of life are also deeply associated with them. The sweetmeat industry is very much integrated into the overall heritage of the culture and have the potentiality to enhance the quality of life style through nutrition and cultural expression. The traditional sweetmeats with their delicious unique flavour, taste, colour and nutrition are essentially based on the regionally available raw materials and the know-how evolved and standardized over 5-7 centuries. However, due to industrial revolution, the various indigenous knowledge are getting eroded due to the fact that these are paying less attention in the present time. Quite a few (sandesh, rosogolla etc.) of the sweetmeats of Bengal have gained the national status and have wider acceptance in abroad (America, Europe, etc.). Most of the traditional techniques are passed on as trade secrets in families, a practice protected by tradition. Although the techniques are primitive, they have played a major role in the economic status of the people. However, complete scientific information on these sweetmeats, their traditional ethics, processing and mode of consumption are lacking. Traditionally some sweetmeats are mostly specific to certain regions depending on the communities. Sweetmeats are mainly prepared from the locally abundantly available raw commodities. In the year 1965 during the period of Prafulla Sen (C.M.) when milk and posset were completely ban in the sweetmeat industry of Kolkata for 1½ year then the sweetmakers were in critical situation. So, they took alternative way and began to prepare herbal sweetmeats from white gourd, bottle gourd, gourd, carrot, coconut, cashewnut, groundnut, pulse-flour, wheat-flour, rice flour, sweet potato, fruit pulp of palmyrah palm, soybean etc. During winter rosogollas' and 'milk rice' are made by palm gur for its peculiar aroma and flavour. Besides palm gur products (*e.g.* sugar, candy, cake, condensed milk, rice milk etc.) are delicious food. The indigenous artisans devoted themselves to get refreshing drinks by tapping the palm trees (Kamble 2003). In the autumn various types of sweetmeats are being made from the fruit pulp of palmyrah palm (*e.g.* sandesh, rosogolla, malpoa, bondey, rosbora, rice, milk etc.).

Materials and Methods

The study was conducted during 1995-2002 covering different localities of W. Bengal. Several visits were made to different parts of the various districts at fortnightly intervals particularly during September to June. During field visits, information on traditional technical knowledge on processing of sweetmeats were also collected through oral interviews with proprietors and employees of the said industries. To fulfill the objectives, study has been conducted in the famous sweetmeat areas. The traditional sweetmeats prepared and presented in the W. Bengal were evaluated based on the criteria of total number of recipe prepared, taste, colour, appearance, flavour nutritional value, degree of traditionalism. Adopting the participatory method involving in different regions did the evaluation of traditional sweetmeats in the recipe contests. After the ensured consent of knowledge holders that knowledge can be put in the public domain through publication. It will facilitate to sustain and preserve the knowledge and institutions related to traditional sweetmeats.

In the preparation of beverage like Haria (rice beer) and Mahua, Bakarh tablets play an important role, act as yeast starter or fermentor which are the mixture of roots, barks, leaves of 5-6 plant species (roots of *Bombax ceiba, Hemidesmus indicus* and *Scoparia dulcis,* stem barks of *Holarrhena pubescens;* leaves of *Buchanania lanzan;* seeds of *Datura metel*) and binded with rice flour. The roots, barks, leaves and seeds are sun dried, powdered and mixed with rice flour in 1 : 2 ratio to make tablets (Kumar and Rao 2007).

Results and Discussion

Almost all people of Bengal are fond of sweetmeats and beverages and consume during every ceremony, festivals, marriages, funeral feasts and sometime offer it to their Gods and deities. Among the beverages, which they consume as cooling and refreshing drinks usually in summer are prepared from various parts of plant species such as *Aegle marmelos* fruit pulp, *Asparagus racemosus* root powder, *Mangifera indica* fruit pulp, *Saccharum officinarum* stem juice, toddy from Palmyrah palm (*Borassus flabellifer*), Date palm (*Phoenix dactylifera, P. sylvestris*), *Madhuca indica* dried corollas, *Oryza saliva* grains (Haria) etc. Each sweetmeats and beverages have great importance in the social life of Bengalees. Sometimes 'Haria' is used to treat fever, dysentery, diarrhoea and gynaecological problems (Sinku 1999) and 'Mahua' and 'Toddy' is given to treat dysentery and diarrhoea. 'Bakarh' tablets are also used to treat cholera. Lukewarm 'Rasogolla's and 'Jilapi' usually used to treat dysentery. The sweetmeats made from the 'pulp of palmyrah palm' are laxative. Though sweetmeats of 'palm gur' are costly yet younger generation does not find tapping occupation acceptable, as it is a painstaking job.

The best popular sweetmeat of Bengal is the numerous types of 'sandesh' and then 'rosogolla' which are of 2 types : Spongy and Crispy. In the year 1917, Fedric Pincot—a British told about 'Sandesh'—It is a food for the Gods and the noble race of Bengalees. Besides in the book of "Bengal sweets

(5th ed)" edited by Mrs. J. Halder—"It is on record that when such an enterprising Indian opened a sweetmeat shop in the parts international Exhibition, his hot jilabis were so much in demand that he sold each for a shilling and even then he could not meet the exorbitant demand." From the raw preparation of 'Rosogollas' various types of sweetmeats are being made by adding various types of additives, dyes or sugars such as Danadar, Kesharbhog, Kamalabhog, Roskadam, Golapjam, Kalojam etc. Besides various types of scented and palatable or delicious sweetmeats are being made in winter from 'palm gur (molasses)' such as rosogollas, rice milk, condensed milk, sandesh, sugar plums etc. Poormans' sweetmeats (pantua) made from tuberous roots of *Ipomoea batatas,* fruit pulp of *Borassus flabellifer,* 'cocoons of silkworm'. The business of sweetmeat Industry in Bengal has a peerless status (*i.e.* ten thousand crores whereas in whole India it is twenty thousand crores and also astonishing for tourists and tourism. During the reception of Tansen at Bishnupur Mallaraj Dynasty the famous sweetmeat 'Motychur' was offered him which is prepared from flour of *Buchanania lanzan* are in the verge of extinct.

Table 2

Sl. No.	Sweetmeat Name	Chief Ingredient Used	Name of the District and Places for its availability	Remarks
1.	Buter Mithai	Gram flour	Bankura–Joyrambati	
2.	*Curd*	Milk	Sonamukhi	
3.	*Khai Chur*	Perched rice	Kotalpur	
4.	*Khir patol*	Condensed milk + deseeded patol	Onda	
5.	*Lagambalatika*	Flour	Bishnupur	
6.	*Mecha-sandesh*	Moog flour	Beliatore, (Dharmarajtola)	Endemic
7.	*Motychur*	Piyal (*B. lanzan* or *Vigna catjang*) flour	Bishnupur	–do–
8.	*Nikhuti*	Rice flour	–do–	
9.	*Rosogolla*	Posset	Sonamukhi	Very cheap
10.	*Tanaladoo*	Pulse flour	Joypur	
11.	*Batasa (sugar plums)*	Sugar	Burdwan-Mankar	
12.	*Gopalgolla*	Posset	–do–	
13.	*Kadma*	–do–	–do–	
14.	*Langcha/Noramisti*	–do– + flour + rice flour	Shaktigarh (200 years ago a British assumed that it in made by Langra)	
15.	*Mihidana*	Pulse flour	Sadar	
16.	*Polau*	Scented rice	–do–	
17.	*Sitabhog*	–do–	–do–	
18.	*Til sandesh*	Seeds of *Sesamum indicum*	–do–	
19.	*Balusai*	Flour + posset	Birbhum–Suri	
20.	*Jalajog*	Condensed milk	–do–	

(Contd...)

(Table 2 – Contd...)

Sl. No.	*Sweetmeat Name*	*Chief Ingredient Used*	*Name of the District and Places for its availability*	*Remarks*
21.	*Kalojam*	Posset + flour	–do–	
22.	*Morobba (Jam)*	Pulp of wood apple, pine-apple etc.	–do–	Cheap
23.	*Amritkumbha*	Posset	Calcutta, Bhowanepur	
24.	*Ashubhog*	–do–	–do–	
25.	*Cake sandesh*	–do– + condensed milk	Gariahat	
26.	*Cham cham*	–do–	–do–	
27.	*Chhanar toast*	–do–	Esplanade	
28.	*Dilkhus*	Groundnut	–do–	
29.	*Golapi panrah*	Condensed milk	Shealdah	
30.	*Khesharbhog*	Keshar + Posset	Bagbazar	The Best maker is Paran Modak
31.	*Khirmohan*	Condensed milk + coarse flour	–do–	
32.	*Ledikeni (pantua)*	Posset + flour	–do–	
33.	*Noukavilas*	Posset	–do–	
34.	*Rajbhog*	–do–	–do–	
35.	*Rosmadhuri*	–do–	–do–	
36.	*Rasmalai*	–do– + milk	–do–	The best maker is Nabin Das
37.	*Rosmanjuri*	Posset	–do–	The best maker is Bhim Nag
38.	*Rosogolla*	–do–	–do–	

(Contd...)

(Table 2 – Contd...)

Sl. No.	Sweetmeat Name	Chief Ingredient Used	Name of the District and places for its availability	Remarks
39.	*Sandesh*	–do–	–do–	
40.	*Steam sandesh*	–do–	–do–	–do–
41.	*Tilmodak*	Seeds of *Sesamum indicum*	Darjeeling	
42.	*Bondey*	Pulse flour	Hooghly–Kamarpukur	
43.	*Chitrakut*	Posset + flour	Srirampore	
44.	*Darbesh*	Cashew + condensed milk + pulse flour	–do–	
45.	*Gaja*	Flour	–do–	
46.	*Jalvora*	Posset	Hooghly-Chandan Nagar	
47.	*Monohora*	–do–	Janai	
48.	*Narikel sandesh*	Coconut	Singoor	
49.	*Chatney of Anaros* *Cham cham*	Pine-apple Posset + flour + milk cream	Jalpaiguri Belakoba	
50.	*Kansert*	Posset	Malda-Sadar	
51.	*Rookadamba*	–do– + condensed milk	–do–	
52.	*Rosvora khanja*	Flour	Pakuahat	
53.	*Amriti*	Rice flour + pulse flour	Paschim Medinipur–Daspur	
54.	*Babarshah*	–do– + banana + flour + ghee	Khirpai	Endemic (named after Edward Babar)
55.	*Chandshahi Khanja*	Flour	C.K. Town	Endemic
56.	*Kalakand*	Posset	Ghatal	

(Contd...)

(Table 2 – Contd...)

Sl. No.	*Sweetmeat Name*	*Chief Ingredient Used*	*Name of the District and places for its availability*	*Remarks*
57.	*Kanchagolla*	–do–	Belda	
58.	*Khir kadam*	Posset + condensed milk	Jhargram	
59.	*Khirer gaja*	Posset + flour + condensed milk	Ghatal	
60.	*Khirer chop*	Posset + flour	Midnapore	
61.	*Mugger jilapi*	Moog	Narayangarh	
62.	*Chatney of rosogallo*	Posset	Purba Medinipur-Contai	
63.	*Kaju sandesh*	Cashewnut	–do–	Endemic
64.	*Swarajbhog*	Milk cream + rice	–do–	–do–
	Chanar-murhki	Posset	Nandakumar	–do–
65.	*Chinir-murhki*	Perched rice	Mursidabad-Khagrah	
66.	*Malpoa*	Flour + banana	Berhampore	
67.	*Badami-golla*	Posset	Nadia-Krishnanagar	
68.	*Dedokhanda*	–do–	–do–	
69.	*Gangajal sandesh*	–do–	–do–	
70.	*Kalo sandesh*	–do–	–do–	
71.	*Khirpuli*	–do–	–do–	
72.	*Nora Pantua*	–do– + flour	Ranaghat	
73.	*Rasasar*	Posset	Krishna Nagar	
74.	*Saratakti*	–do–	–do–	
75.	*Sarvaja*	Milk cream	–do–	

(Contd...)

(Table 2 – Contd...)

Sl. No.	*Sweetmeat Name*	*Chief Ingredient Used*	*Name of the District and places for its availability*	*Remarks*
76.	*Sarpuria*	–do–	–do–	Endemic
77.	*Toast sandesh*	Posset	–do–	–do–
78.	*Gupo-sandesh*	–do–	North 24 Parganas-Panihati	–do–
79.	*Jilapi*	Rice flour + pulse flour	Barrackpur	
80.	*Nikhuti*	Posset	Barasat	
81.	*Roskadamba*	–do–	Panihati	
82.	*Sonpapri*	Flour + pulse flour	Kanchrapara	
83.	*Mowa*	Kanakchur dhan	South 24 Parganas-Joynagar	Endemic
84.	*Halua*	Coarse flour	Purulia	
85.	*Murkhi*	Tulaipanji dhan (perched rice)	Uttardinajpur-Balurghat	Endemic
86.	*Khirer Singarah*	Posset + flour	Siliguri	

2.3 Traditional Endemic Gahanabarhis of Purba Medinipur

Abstract

The people in Purba Medinipur (specially in Tamluk sub-division) have a tradition of relishing a variety of barhis, locally called 'gahana barhi' specially prepared during winter months. These little balls are produced from the partially fermentation of black gram (*Phaseolus mungo L*) batters. These products include seeds of *Papaver somniferum L.* and sometimes alongwith various spices which are unknown to the scientific community. This new crispy food is described with respect to the nature of the product, method of preparation, mode of consumption and ethnic value.

Keywords : *Gahanabarhi, Purba Medinipur, Tamluk.*

Introduction

Traditional or indigenous foods are those popular products that since the time immemorial have formed an integral part of the tiffin, curry and that can be prepared in the household industry using relatively simple techniques and equipment (Aidoo *et. al.,* 2006). Fermentation improves pulse digestibility for humans, improved flavour, colour and reduced cooking time. Sometimes pulse paste containing spices and salt, the preserving quality is considerably enhanced. Here the indigenous techniques are passed on as trade secrets in the families of certain communities. Although several legume-based fermented foods like idle, dhosa, papad, pitha etc. from different parts of India have been documented (Roy *et. al.,* 2007) but there is no documentation on gahanabarhi. Gahanabarhi (goina bari) is usually prepared by 'Beulis' in different community blocks of Purba Medinipur (Tamluk, Moyna, Panskura etc.) which is an indigenous popular renowned cottage industry of the self-help group. These 'gahanabarhis' are now receiving world attention for their taste and beauty. It exists for 300 years and praised by renowned persons like Abanindranath Tagore, Ramananda Chattopadhyay, Jaladhar Sen, Rabindranath Tagore, Nandalal Basu, Satyajit Roy etc. Therefore, the objective of this survey was to look for cheaply available legume-based peculiar charming food. Generally the cost of locally available dehusked seeds of black gram varies from Rs. 35-40 kg.

Materials and Methods

A survey was conducted in the different villages of Tamluk subdivision under the district Purba Medinipur during winter of the year 2001 to obtain detailed information on gahanabarhi, their traditional method of preparation. For the preparation a thick handkerchief alongwith a stitched button like round perforation in the centre is required. A both side opened hollow conical metal pipe (length 1") may be easily fasten or fixed in the central perforation of the cloth. In a word the combination of pipe and the cloth is called "Chong-putli." To prepare the 'gahanabarhi', 1 kg biri kalai, (black gram *Phaseolus mungo L.*) seeds are soaked for overnight in the cold water for dehusking. In the morning of the next day at 8–9 am the dehusked black gram seeds are made into a paste with the help of a grinding stone and add a spoonful of edible salt. To assist the chief artisan a helper or amplifier is required who will add the requisite amount of water in the paste and repeatedly amplify (beat up into froth) the paste with the help of hand at different angles to give it buoyancy. In the mean time the amplified paste is fell down by the chief artisan through the Chong-putli on the scattered poppy seeds in the oily tray or plate to get a desired design (such as necklace, bracelet, ear-drop, crown, conch-shell etc.). The helper supply the paste to the chief artisan as and when required. The barhis are of different types *e.g.* topa, bichey, amriti, jilapi etc. Of them skilled hand is essential to prepare gahanabarhi. To achieve coloured gahanabarhis desirable vegetable dyes can be mixed in the paste. From 1 kg gram seeds 150 pieces of 'gahanabarhis' can be made. Now the trays containing raw barhis will be placed in the direct sunlight consecutively for 2–3 days for easy procuration and proper drying.

Results and Discussion

This ornamental delicious easily digestible fast food is

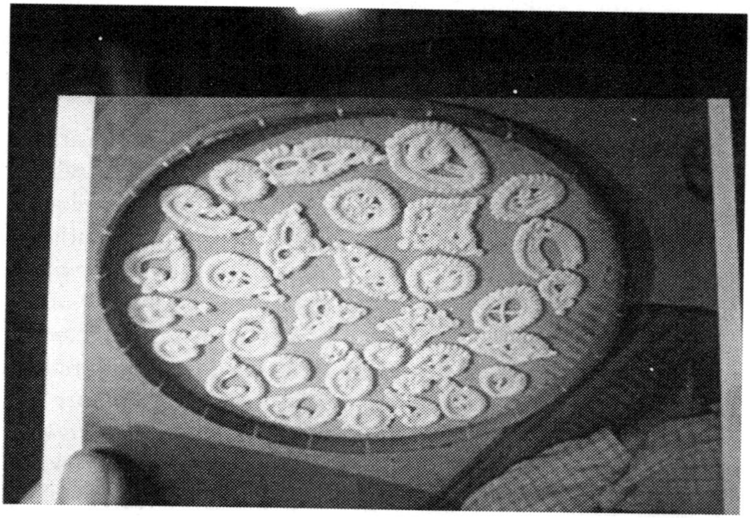

Various Designs of Barhis

popularly used as tiffin round the year through instant frying. Besides these barhis are consumed by all the communities irrespective of caste and creed in curry, soup, sour etc. Someone used these barhis to decorate their drawing room which lasts for a year. The remarkable designs of barhis (such as sitahar, sitadul, chiruni, lalantika, lockehar, konkon, mukut, joraful etc.) are very lucrative and can be presented for exhibition in the Art School. The humidity alongwith cloudy or foul weather is the chief enemy for the barhis. So, frequent direct sun drying is necessary to keep the barhis well. Generally all the artisans (beulis) are the women. The taste of the barhis enhanced with the advent of winter as at that time weather is relatively dry and decreased in the rainy season in contact with humidity. At present in these localities bed-tea or breakfast is served with frying palatable gahanabarhis instead of biscuits, snacks or papad which focuses the aristocracy of this type of tiffin. The net profit of an artisan by preparing 1 Kg of gahanabarhis is near about one hundred rupees. To keep the relation concrete with relatives this presentable food stuff can be compared with sweetmeats.

2.4 Home Made Amusing Diabetic Food

Water chestnut (Bull's head) grown abundantly in the ponds, swamps and ditches of Bengal during the winter months. A nutritious low caloric self made diabetic food called singarha flour is produced by village women of Purba Medinipur, West Bengal for domestic and marketing purposes. It is healthful, sugar free and contains low percentage of carbohydrate for the good growth of Juvenile diabetic patients.

For preparing amusing Singarha flour good quality water chestnut (*Trapa bispinosa* L, Hydrocaryaceae) (Bengali-Pani Phal, Hindi-Singarha) and green gram, *Vigna radiata* (Linn) are taken in 3:1 ratio. They are washed and dried in sunlight then roasted separately and mixed. The mixed edible parts are then grinded and stored in packets. It is cheaper and supplied by self-supporting womens groups in the villages of Purba Medinipur like Panskura, Kolaghat, etc. Flour of Singarha is now gradually become a popular food among the aged people also as it is rich in nutrients and ideally suited to the physical conditions. Due to the increasing cost of prepared proteinaceous foods it is necessary to look for other cheap and non-conventional source of food. This food is particularly profitable for poors, bakery industry and sweet makers as an alternative source of wheat.

2.5 Wild Edible Plants of West Rarrh

Abstract

The tribals are in close association with nature and largely depends on forest product for their livelihood. As a result they acquired a vast knowledge about wild plants. The wild plants are playing a vital role in providing nutritional and revenue earning security to the poor aboriginals. But still many of them are neglected and never documented for their ethnobotanical importance. Keeping in mind an ethnobotanical survey was performed to collect, identify and document information on the wild food plants traditionally used by the tribals.

Keywords : *Wild edible plants, Ethnobotany, West Rarrh.*

Introduction

Wild plants provide food and other life-supporting commodities. Besides they maintain the ecological balance. Generally forests are the main reservoir of biodiversity as they harbour of about 50% of the total species. Forests have a prominent role for improving food security of forest dwellers. In India, about 550 tribal communities contribute 8.08% of the total population. Tribals are well acquainted with the plants of surrounding forests and knew what to eat and how to separate harmful substances from the edible part of plants such as to remove raphides of elephant leg and *Dioscorea* they at first peeled it, boiled in tamarind water and smeared with turmeric paste or the peeled are sun-dried for few days. West Rarrh is located at 21°75′ to 24°33′ N latitude and 85°70′ to 87°80′E longitude. The geographical area of West Rarrh is about 27,500 sq.km of which 35% constitute forest.

In West Bengal certain wild tuber, rhizome, root, leaf, flower, fruit, legumes including tribal pulses are consumed by the tribals (Jain 1981, 1991). Generally in West Bengal tribals constitute an important component representing about 8% of the total population of India. But in West Rarrh it is about 9% of the total population of West Bengal. There are at least 3000 edible plant species known to man, with merely 30 crops contributing to more than 90% of the world's calorie intake, and only 120 crops are economically significant at national level.

The study highlights some of the important wild food plants, which need to be documented for food security in future.

Tribals lives in forest ecosystem and have their own traditional food habits as settled agriculture does not provide them sufficient food due to non fertile land. So, they largely depend on wild food to supplement their staple food. The range of these types of foods used by the tribals varies from locality to locality depending on tribal types.

Methodology

Field survey was carried out during the period between

1995 to 2005. At each time of visit, different tribal hamlets and forest pockets were chosen in different seasons to collect more information. The information was accrued by repeated interviews through questionnaires based on the information provided by the tribals. The plant specimens were identified by the taxonomist (Dr. Manindranath Sanyal) and the prepared herbarium sheets (Jain and Rao 1967); were kept in the Dept. of Botany, Bishnupur Ramananda College, Bankura.

Results and Discussion

Wild plants belonging to 55 families (5 gymnosperm) being eaten by different tribals of W. Rarrh have been tabulated alphabetically with plant named/s), family, vernacular name(s) and plant parts used (Table 3). Of the various parts, tribals consume rhizome, corms, tubers, bulbils and root types of 13 plant species; stem pith and apical meristems of 11 plant species; leaves of 31 plant species; flowers of 3 plants species; fruits of 38 plant species; seeds, endosperm and kernels of 5 plant species. The plant parts are eaten either raw or cooked form. Among the documented edible plant species of W. Rarrh 7 species (*Flacourtia indica, Gymnema sylvestre, Ipomoea digitata, Syzygium jambos, Syzygium samarangense, Terminalia catappa, Ziziphus oenoplia*) are listed in threatened category. So, suitable conservation techniques should be followed to preserve them for future generations as such edible wild plants also act as supplementary food during lean and stress period. Besides these plants not only help in relieving ailments but also fetch sometimes a good market price. Therefore, sustainable management of biodiversity is essential. There is much scope for improving the food processing techniques for the edible wild plants to make them acceptable recipes.

Table 3

Sl.No.	Botanical Name	Vernacular Name	Family	Habit	Edible Part
1.	*Abrus precatorius* L.	Kunch	Fabaceae	Tree	Leaf
2.	*Achras zapota* L.	Safeda	Sapotaceae	–do–	Fruit
3.	*Adhatoda vasica Nees.*	Basak	Acanthaceae	Shrub	Leaf
4.	*Aegle marmelos* (L.) Corr.	Bel	Rutaceae	Tree	Fruit, Leaf
5.	*Aerva lanata* (L.) Juss	Daya phul	Amaranthaceae	Herb	Tender leaf
6.	*Alangium salviifolium* (L.f.) Wong.	Ankar	Alangiaceae	Tree	Fruit
7.	*Alternanthera sessilis* (L.) DC.	Sincheshak	Amaranthaceae	Herb	Leaf
8.	*Amaranthus spinosus* L.	Kantanotey	–do–	–do–	–do–
9.	*Anacardium occidentale* L.	Kaju badam	Anacardiaceae	Shrub	Pericarp
10.	*Artocarpus lakoocha* Roxb.	Madar	Moraceae	Tree	Fruit
11.	*Annona squamosa* L.	Ata	Annonaceae	Shrub	–do–
12.	*A. reticulata* L.	Nona	–do–	–do–	–do–
13.	*Asparagus racemosus* Willd.	Satamuli	Liliaceae	Under shrub	Root
14.	*Averrhoa carambola* L.	Kamranga	Oxalidaceae	Tree	Fruit
15.	*Bacopa monnieri* L.	Brahmi	Scrophulariaceae	Creeper	Leaf
16.	*Bambusa arundinacea* (Retz.)	Bans	Poaceae	Herb	Young shoot
17.	*Bixa orellana* L.	Lotkon	Bixaceae	Shrub	Fruit
18.	*Boerhavia diffusa* L.	Punarnaba	Nyctaginaceae	Herb	Leaf

(Contd...)

(Table 3 – Contd...)

Sl.No.	Botanical Name	Vernacular Name	Family	Habit	Edible Part
19.	*Buchanania lanzan* Spreng.	Piyal	Anacardiaceae	Tree	Fruit
20.	*Butea monosperma* (Lamk.) Taub.	Palash	Fabaceae	–do–	Young roots for bread
21.	*Centella asiatica* (L.)	Thankuni	Apiaceae	Herb	Leaf
22.	*Celosia argentea* L.	Muragjhuti	Amaranthaceae	–do–	Tender shoot
23.	*Cephalandra indica* Naud.	Telakuncha	Cucurbitaceae	–do–	Leaf, green fruit
24.	*Ceratopteris thalictroides*	Dhenki Shak	Parkeriaceae	Aquatic fern	Leaf
25.	*Chenopodium album* L.	Bethoshak	Chenopodiaceae	Herb	–do–
26.	*Cleome viscosa* L.	Hoorhuria	Capparidaceae	–do–	Tender shoot
27.	*Cannabis sativa* L.	Ganja	Cannabinaceae	Shrub	Leaf/Inflorescence
28.	*Carissa carandas* L.	Karamcha	Apocynaceae	–do–	Sour fruits
29.	*C. spinarum* L.	Karowan	–do–	–do–	Fruit
30.	*Carthamus tinctorius* L.	Kusum	Asteraceae	Herb	Seed
31	*Cassia tora* L.	Chakunda	Caesalpiniaceae	Shrub	Leaf
32.	*Colocasia esculenta* (L.) Schott.	Kachu	Araceae	Herb	Petiole, Rhizome
33.	*Commelina benghalensis* L.	Dholapata/Kanshira	Commelinaceae	–do–	Leaf
34.	*Corchorus capsularis* L.	Titapat	Tiliaceae	–do–	–do–
35.	*C. olitorius* L.	Pat	–do–	–do–	–do–
36.	*Curculigo orchioides* Gaertn.	Talamuli/Musali	Amaryllidaceae	–do–	Rhizome

(Contd...)

(Table 3 – Contd...)

Sl.No.	Botanical Name	Vernacular Name	Family	Habit	Edible Part
37.	*Curcuma longa* L.	Halud	Zingiberaceae	–do–	–do–
38.	*Cyperus rotundus* L.	Muthaghas	Cyperaceae	–do–	Tuberous root
39.	*Dillenia indica* L.	Chalta	Dilleniaceae	Tree	Calyx
40.	*Dioscorea pentaphylla* L.	Khamalu	Dioscoreaceae	Twiner	Tuber
41.	*Diospyros exsculpta* Buch. Ham	Kend	Ebenaceae	Tree	Fruit
42.	*Dryopteris filix-mas*	Shield fern	Polypodiaceae	Herb	Tender shoot
43.	*Emblica officinalis* Gaertn.	Amlaki	Euphorbiaceae	Tree	Fruit
44.	*Enhydra fluctuans* Lour.	Hingcha	Asteraceae	Herb	Leaf
45.	*Euryale ferox Salish*	Makhna	Nymphaeaceae	Aquatic herb	Seed
46.	*Feronia elephantum* Corr.	Kaith	Rutaceae	Tree	Fruit
47.	*Ficus carica* L.	Dumur	Moraceae	–do–	–do–
48.	*Flacourtia indica* (Burm. F.)	Bainchi	Flacourtiaceae	Shrub	–do–
49.	*Gymnema sylvestre* W. and A.	Gulmur	Asclepiadaceae	Woody climber	Leaf
50.	*Hemidesmus indicus* (L.) R. Br.	Anantamul	–do–	Prostrate shrub	Root bark
51.	*Holoptela integrifolia* (Roxb.) Planch	Chhalla	Ulmaceae	Tree	Fruit
52.	*Hygrophila auriculata* (Schum.) Heine	Kulekhara	Acanthaceae	Herb	Leaf
53.	*Ipomoea aquatica* Forssk.	Kalmi	Convolvulaceae	Aquatic herb	Leaf
54.	*I. batatas* (L.) Lamk.	Rangalu	–do–	Trailing herb	Tuberous root
55.	*I. digitata* L.	Bhui kumra	–do–	Climber	–do–

(Contd...)

(*Table 3 – Contd...*)

Sl.No.	*Botanical Name*	*Vernacular Name*	*Family*	*Habit*	*Edible Part*
56.	*Leonotis nepetifolia* L.	Agni-janum	Lamiaceae	Herb	Young twig
57.	*Maranta arundinacea* L.	Araroot	Marantaceae	–do–	Rhizome
58.	*Madhuca indica* Gmel	Mahua	Sapotaceae	Tree	Fruit
59.	*Marselia quadrifolia* L.	Susni	Marseliaceae	Aquatic herb	Leaf
60.	*Mentha arvensis* L.	Pudina	Lamiaceae	Herb	–do–
61.	*Mimusops elengi* L.	Bakul	Sapotaceae	Tree	Ripe fruit
62.	*Mirabilis jalapa* L.	Sandhyamoni	Nyctaginaceae	Erect herb	Ripe fried seed
63.	*Morus alba* L.	Tunt	Moraceae	Tree	Fruit
64.	*Murraya koenigii* (L.) Spreng	Currypata	Rutaceae	Shrub	Leaf
65.	*Nelumbo nucifera Gaertn*	Padma	Nymphaeaceae	Floating herb	Carpel
66.	*Nephelium longana* (Lamk.) Camb	Anshphal	Sapindaceae	Tree	Aril
67.	*Nymphaea nouchali* Burm. f.	Shalook	Nymphaeaceae	Aquatic herb	Seed
68.	*Oryza rufipogon* Griff.	Basudhan	Poaceae	Herb	Grain
69.	*Oxalis corniculata* L.	Amrul	Oxaalidaceae	Procumbent	Leaf
70.	*Pachyrhizus angulatus* Rich.	Shakalu	Fabaceae	Climber	Tuberos root
71.	*Paederia foetida* L.	Gendhal	Rubiaceae	Twining shrub	Leaf
72.	*Papaver somniferum* L.	Afinggach	Papaveraceae	Herb	Seed/resin
73.	*Passiflora foetida* L.	Jhumkalata	Passifloraceae	Climber	Ripe fruit

(*Contd...*)

(Table 3 – Contd...)

Sl.No.	Botanical Name	Vernacular Name	Family	Habit	Edible Part
74.	*Pennisetum typhoides* Burm. f.	Bajra	Poaceae	Tall herb	Grain
75.	*Phoenix acaulis* Buch.	Ban khejur	Arecaceae	Tree	Fruit
76.	*P. sylvestris* (L.) Roxb	Khejur	–do–	–do–	–do–
77.	*Piper betle* L.	Pan	Piperaceae	Climber	Leaf
78.	*P. longum* L.	Pipul	–do–	–do–	Fruit
79.	*Polypodium decorum*	Polypodium	Polypodiaceae	Herb	Leaf
80.	*Portulaca oleracea* L.	Lunia-shak	Portulacaceae	–do–	–do–
81.	*Pteris longifolia*	–do–	Polypodiaceae	–do–	–do–
82.	*Psidium guajava* L.	Peyara	Myrtaceae	Tree	Fruit
83.	*Ruellia tuberosa* L.	Kalo phatka	Acanthaceae	Herb	Tuberous root
84.	*Schleichera oleosa* (Lour) Oken	Kusum	Sapindaceae	Tree	Aril
85.	*Semecarpus anacardium* L.	Bhelai	Anacardiaceae	–do–	Pericarp/cotyledon
86.	*Sesbania grandiflora* Pers.	Bakphul	Fabaceae	Climber	Flower
87.	*Spondias pinnata* (L.) Kurz.	Amrah	–do–	Tree	Fruit
88.	*Streblus asper* Lour.	Sheorah	Moraceae	–do–	Ripe fruit
89.	*Syzygium cumini* (L.) Skeels	Kalojam	Myrtaceae	–do–	Fruit
90.	*S. jambos* (L.) *Aalston*	Gulabjam	–do–	–do–	–do–
91.	*S. samarangense* (Blume)	Jamrul	–do–	–do–	–do–
92.	*Terminalia catappa* L.	Jangli-badam	Combretaceae	–do–	Nut

(Contd...)

(Table 3 – Contd...)

Sl.No.	Botanical Name	Vernacular Name	Family	Habit	Edible Part
93.	*Tamarindus indica* L.	Tentul	Caesalpiniaceae	–do–	Fruit
94.	*Trapa bispinosa* (Roxb.) Makino	Paniphal	Trapaceae	Aquatic herb	–do–
95.	*Tridax procumbens* L.	Tridaksha	Asteraceae	Herb	Leaf
96.	*Vangueria spinosa* Roxb.	Moinakanta	Rubiaceae	Shrub	Fruit
97.	*Vigna catjang* (Burm. f.)	Barbati	Fabaceae	Climber	Pod
98.	*Zea mays* L.	Janar	Poaceae	Tall herb	Grains
99.	*Ziziphus jujuba* Mill.	Kul	Rhamnaceae	Tree	Fruit
100.	*Z. oenoplia*	Shiakul	–do–	Straggling Shrub	–do–

2.6 How One Can Achieve Desire Qualities of Honey from Detached Apiphilic Plants for Health Care in the Off-Season

Abstract

It focuses on Indian traditional knowledge (ITK), innovation practices and beliefs pertaining to honey industry and is being used therapeutically. Frequently honey is being produced from detached plant part in off seasons mixed in sugar solution instead of any loss of worker bees in Natures' calamity. The study deals with instant food making process of bees.

Keywords : *Apiphilic, Paanchamrita, Palynology, Unifloral, Bee flora.*

Introduction

Honey gives life to the mankind. So, since time immemorial Indian priests used to mix honey in Panchamrita, a sacred liquid-mixture served to the human in worship place for a long time. In India *Nymphaea rubra* (lotus) honey is used for opthalmic diseases. *Ocimum basilicum, O. sanctum* honey is used for cough, sore throats, earache and in gastric ulcers. Recent studies also reveals that honey from tulsi is a best remedy for peptic ulcer. No adverse effect of honey have been reported till now. Besides honey is the best tropical medicine for the healing of wounds both in human and veterinary. Honey cleans the wound without any surgical interference. Honey reduces inflammation, stimulates healing process, hastens tissue regeneration. No product made by man can mimic honey made by bees. Honey production varies with the quality and quantity of nectar present in different flowering plants. Bees also never like all the plants for taking nectar. They generally select the bright coloured and scented flowers having sufficient nectar. The essential raw materials of honey are nectar and pollen grains. Bees often, intend to collect nectar from single species, if such species is found abundant in a particular area. In natural process quality of honey is determined by its palynoassemblage and palyno-assemblage depends on the floral fidelity of the worker bees, which further reveals the bee flora of an area.

Materials and Methods

For the management of bees and getting more honey by instant process in the off seasons (in rainy and autumn) bee-keepers may well acquainted with this process. To get particular quality of honey the flower or leaf extract of that particular plant may be added to the sugar solution. A flower or leaf extract to attract bees is prepared and processed with sugar solution (100 g sugar + 1 litre water), flower/leaf extract (25g) and 1 drop kerosene oil. This will be the artificial regular diet for 25 bee keeping boxes to accustomed with the particular plant product in the off-season and to create a general affinity for the bees. Honey samples have been kept in the palynology laboratory for testing the medicated value. Locally available plants are used for honey. The data has been accrued for traditional food and therapy followed by 3 consecutive years.

Results and Discussions

This finding may provide new sources of honey in off-season when profuse flowers are lacking. The formulation of these effective phyto-solutions should be encouraged the bee-keepers for their sustainable uses. To meet the particular demand of honey according to the requirement of ailment this honey making process is effective and at the same time it prevents the loss of bees as there is no need for pollen collection in the clumsy days. In this practice 'Unifloral honey is being made which is usually distinct in colour, flavour and taste.

Bee-beverage yielding process has been carried out especially on considering the food value, its medical efficacy as well as on market value and on economic importance.

Still in West Bengal, such studies have not got much attention of the apiculturist inspite of having a good potentiality of apiculture.

Some plants suitable for this practice has been enumerated below :

1. Storage root extract of *Daucus carota*. This honey prevents the eye diseases.

2. Petal extract of *Rosa centifolia*. This honey is suitable for skin care.
3. Leaf extract of *Ocimum basilicum, O. sanctum*. This honey is suitable against cough, cold, sore throat, peptic ulcer etc.
4. Leaf and flower extract of *Psydium guajava and Psyzigium cumini*. This honey is used for diabetic drink.
5. Flower extract of *Nymphaea rubra*. This honey is effective for eye diseases.

2.7 Abolishing Traditional Pithas (Cakes) of Bengal

Abstract

The people of Bengal have a tradition of relishing a variety of cakes, locally called pitha, specially prepared during 'Makar Sankranti', in various rituals and during winter months. The study describes the traditional pithas of indigenous people of Bengal and documented them for the welfare of cake-lovers before being abolishing. As a result the pottery, native paddy varieties and husking-pedals will be preserved from the verge of extinction. The study gives an overview of the history, current status, problems and prospects of pithas industry in Bengal.

Keywords : *Traditional pitha, Palm Gur, Tapper artisans, West Rarrh, Tushu Parav.*

Introduction

Traditional or indigenous foods are those popular products, that since early history have formed an integral part of the diet and that can be made in the household or in cottage industry using relatively simple techniques and equipment (Aidoo *et. al.,* 2006). Many pithas of Bengal are now receiving world attention for their delicacy, flavour, nutritional value and appearance. Some ethnic groups of Bengal are habituated with these popular varieties of pithas during winter months. Some techniques of pitha making are passed on as trade secrets in the families of certain communities, a practice protected by tradition

(Taming *et. al.*, 1988). Although several legume-based pithas, like idli, dosa etc. have been well studied and scaled-up but there is no documentation on pitha-diversity of rural-bengal which may help the self-supporting groups to develop and also to earn money like the sweetmeat industry.

During 20th century in Bengal a bride can be adjudged or selected on her pitha making ability. It was a staple food in the age of Vedic. Though then the pithas were made from barley (job). Pithas made from rice was started at the end of Rig Veda. So the age of pithas are of near about 1,500 B.C. and it is evolved from Eastern Countries. There are numerous names about pithas like Pupa, Apupa, Apupic, Pista, Puradash, Papat, Sajjuli, Khenak, Laddur, Ghritapur, Madhumastaka etc. In ancient time sacrifice festival, funeral ceremony and festival of eating new rice could not be executed without pitha and palmgur. So it can easily be assumed that during the age of Purana (the ancient mythology of Hindus) pitha was an integral part of cultural status of Bengalee. The bard, the follower of Vishnu, Sri Krishna and Sri Ramakrishna likes the so called pithas. The famous artist Mirabye sacrificed the 'Gokulpitha' in the honour of Sri Krishna.

Materials and Methods

A survey was performed during winter in the different pockets of rural areas throughout West Bengal since 1999 as the villages are the chief source for this type of cottage industry. Where husking pedals, clay pots and different varieties of paddy are available. During this survey a detailed information on the types, traditional method of preparation, modes of consumption etc. has been collected for pithas. Rural grandmothers are making the showy ornamented tasty pithas with the help of rice-flour, pulse flour, milk, coconut, molasses, condensed milk etc. in the clay images and clay cake-basket. Some of the remarkable pithas of Bengal are Chitoi, Saruchakuli, Askey, Gokulpitha, Purpitha, Partysapta, Harshepur, Chandrapuli, Rospuli, Gurpitha, Dudhpuli, Shahipuli, Poapitha (pana pitha),

Rosbora, Talbora, Malpoa, Dhukipitha, Jantalpitha, Rangalupitha etc. Some are described below :

(*i*) **Saru Chakuli :** Which resembles dosa, is a thin and round fried pancake. It is prepared from varying proportions of par-boiled rice and black gram (*Phaseolus mungo* L.). Black gram may be substituted with juice of jackfruit or palmyra palm fruit pulp or pounded kernel or Mahua flower or bottle gourd. At first rice is washed, soaked for overnight, dewatered through a perforated bowl and sun-dried. Dried rice grains are pounded in a wooden husking pedal or mortar and sieved to obtain a fine powder. Black gram is also soaked for overnight until the seed-coat is easily removable by applying a mild pressure. After the black gram is made into a paste using a stone grinder. The paste is beaten repeatedly by hands with a little amount of fresh water and mixed with rice flour, required amount of lukewarm water and edible salt. The batter is then spreading and fried over a hot oily pan to round shaped flat cake. Spices, like ginger, onion, black pepper, cardamom powder are sometimes added at the time of frying for enhancing the taste. The shelf life of chakuli pitha is only one day. It is eaten with curry, palmgur, lukewarm milk.

(*ii*) **Partysapta Pitha :** The preparation method is similar to that of saru chakuli pitha. At first the flattening of batter over a hot oily pan using a spatula then the fillings of grated coconut, chhana and molasses are taken in the centre of the pancake followed by folding. It has a shelf life of 2 days and is usually eaten without any adjunct.

(*iii*) **Tal Gangra :** Batter is prepared by blending of rice powder with the fruit pulp of Palmyra palm (*Borassus flabellifer*) and then minced. After it is fried on 'open pan' containing sufficient amount of boiling oil. Their shelf life is 2-3 days and is eaten with or without adjunct.

(*iv*) **Ol Pitha :** Batter is prepared by blending of dehusked sun-dried Ol (corm) powder (*Amorphophallus campanu-*

latus) with rice powder and then minced. Then it is fried on greasy open pan.

(*v*) **Tal Bora :** Batter is prepared by blending of wheat flour with the fruit pulp of palmyra palm and then minced. Then it is fried on greasy open pan.

(*vi*) **Pata Pitha :** It is a steamed flavoured cake, prepared by taking the fermented batter (as prepared in making Saru chakuli) in a banyan leaf and folding the leaf through mid-vein. It may also be stuffed with coconut, chhana and sugar fillings. The batter-filled folded leaves are then boiled over steam. Its shelf-life is 2 days and is usually may be eaten without any adjunct.

(*vii*) **Pana Pitha :** For the preparation of pana pitha, fermented batter (as performed in making chakuli) is mixed with small pieces of (minced) coconut, ground nut, cashew nut and sugar. The mixture is covered or packed by banana leaf. The packets are then covered around by hot charcoal in an earthen oven to bake in low but continuous heat for 5-6 hrs at night. In the next morning, the product is cut into pieces and served. Its shelf-life is 3-4 days and may be eaten without adjunct.

(*viii*) **Purpitha :** Fine powder of rice mixed with boiled water (sometimes blended with palmyra palm pulp) and made into paste and then minced. The centre of each piece is stuffed with coconut or sesame or chhana or condensed milk and sugar filling. Sufficient water is taken in a handi (large mouthed vessel), for boiling and a perforated pitcher containing pieces of pithas is placed over the handi for cooking in the steam.

(*ix*) **Anskey Pitha :** It is prepared by mixing the fermented batter (as prepared in making Saru Chakuli). It is then taken in a special earthen mould or in a bowl and covered with a lid. The junction is closed with a wet cloth and water is sprinkled intermittently. It is fried on a mild heat to make it spongy. It is generally taken with curry, palm gur etc.

(*x*) **Gur Pitha :** Batter is prepared by blending of rice powder with milk and molasses. Then it is fried on open pan containing sufficient amount of boiling oil. Its shelf life is 2 days and is eaten without adjunct.

(*xi*) **Rangalu Pitha :** Wheat flour is mixed with boiled dehusked sweet potato and made into paste and then minced. The centre of each pieces is stuffed with coconut, cashewnut, condensed milk, poppy seeds and sugar filling. Then all the pieces are fried in ghee to achieve light red in colour and soaked for 3 hrs in sugar juice. Its shelf life is 3 days and is eaten without adjunct.

(*xii*) **Gokul Pitha :** Batter is prepared by blending of wheat flour in cold milk and then minced. The centre of each piece is stuffed with cardamom, coconut, ground nut, condensed milk. Then all the pieces are fried in ghee and soaked for 3 hrs in sugar juice. Its shelf life is 2-3 days and is eaten without adjunct.

Results and Discussion

As all these pithas are delicious and easily digestible in winter months so popularly consumed by all the communities irrespective of caste and creed in 'Makar Sankranti' alongwith palm gur. Without palm gur and pitha-puli Bengalee culture can not be imaginated during winter. Due to advances in rapid industrialization, civilization alongwith sophistication the Bengals' folk culture like pitha-puli and festival of eating new rice with palm gur is gradually being diminishing. Besides due to hazardous nature of work alongwith rapid depletion of date-palm the newly made treacle from date-palm is gradually being abolishing. The making of golden palm gur with its characteristic aroma and flavour is one of the shinning traditional skills of Bengals tappers during the winter months. The indigenous artisans, for ages are engaged in the tapping palmyra palm and date palm to get sweet neera which ultimately gives gut or jaggery are the integral part of pitha-puli. Tree climbing process for tapping palm trees still remains though it is the most difficult and arduous task at the dawn of winter.

It provides employment to the artisans for 3-4 months in a year. Though pithas are made more or less in various festivals throughout the year but it is intensified in 'Makar Sankranti'. So it is called pitha parav. It can provides employment to the rural artisans with meagre financial investment. It has a very good prospect and market in Bengal due to its uniqueness. Rice and Pulse flour processing were traditionally done manually by beating the heavy wooden husking pedals or by grinding stone. Recently flour processing machine have been introduced. In West Bengal still 48 scented varieties of rice are existing. Of them Sonamukhi, Laxshmibhog, Gobindabhog, Kartickshal etc. are the best for achieving the scented pithas. Pitha fair is now started in 10th January 2009 at Prembazar of Kharagpur and in Digha.

Due to lack of fond of work or untiring worker alogwith rapid expansion of education the younger woman generation from rural areas does not find this cottage industry acceptable, as it is not adequately remunerative. To revive the pithas cordiality is the first and foremost or fundamental element. The pithas, the time–honoured precepts and the household food should not be enduring in the hand of greedy commercialist if proper precaution is not taken. Still in West Rarrh of Bengal Tushu Parav (festival) and pitha-puli is complementary to each other in 'Makar Sankranti'. An extensive research in the field of pitha industry is required to develop and popularise the cake in different festivals.

The production of these pithas has remained a traditional village art practiced in homes in a crude manner. Due to dealing of fast life there is a gradual inclination of the younger generation of the villages towards the modern fast foods, under-estimating their own indigenous pithas. These household blending processes are complicated and time wastaging. Hence many of them are being replaced by industrially processed pithas. Besides indigenous processings are not always ideal and scientific. So, there is need for further research for its improvement.

2.8 Indigenous Knowledge on Various Fruit Pulp Processing of Suri in Birbhum District of West Bengal

Abstract

Indigenous technical knowledge (ITK) on the processing of Fruit pulp of various plants has been communicated for income generating and nutrient supplementation. Fruit sellers normally process the fruits for their household business as jam, jelly etc. by crushing and boiling the fruits, whereas entrepreneurs purchase the fruits from growers and produces 18 varieties of edible pulp cake indigenously called Morobba for selling in the market of Suri as well as in neighbouring districts of W. Bengal.

***Keywords** : Fruit pulp processing, Morobba, Suri.*

Introduction

The Birbhum district is situated between the 23°23′30′′ and 24°25′ latitude. The eastern most extremity of the district is marked by 88°01′40′′ E longitude and its western most extremely by 87°05′25′′ N. The district Head Quarter is Suri. It has been found that various indigenous knowledge to procure Morobba are being practiced since 300 years ago. Morobba preparation can help the growers to prevent the deterioration of the fruits. Suri is unique for processing and utilization of different types of fruits. Morobbas are usually prepared from the ripened fruit pulp which are very popular throughout W. Bengal in off season. Fruit products are presently consumed mostly within the country but have potential for international market promotion (Chhetri and Gauchan 2007).

Materials and Method

The study was performed at fortnightly intervals during winter months in the session 2001-02 covering throughout Suri which is famous for traditional Morobba. At the time of field survey information on pulp processing to procure Morobba from different types of matured fruit pulp was collected through conversation among the workers engaged in processing this type of cottage industry. Interrogation has emphasized the harvesting techniques, categories and mode of trading of fruits.

Results and Discussion

Generally seasonal fruit harvesting takes place in their matured condition just before ripening for pulp processing. As a result Morobba can easily preserved for 1-2 years and be used to treat different ailments throughout the year even when the particular fruit is not available in the market. To enhance the durability of Morobba the matured fruits are harvested during Sunny days at noon and proper precaution will be taken during pulp processing alongwith their preservation technique. Normally fruit processing is done at commercial, semi-commercial and in domestic scale. Sometimes farmers sell their fruits directly to local processors at their farmyard or orchard. Though some farmers process it for their household needs as sauce, whereas entrepreneurs purchase the fruits from growers and process different varieties of Morobba for marketing commercially in India and Abroad. There are nearly 18 varieties of Morobba being processed in Suri. The common steps involved in processing the fruit pulps are mentioned here :

At first wash the desired fruits to remove dirt and dehusked where the rind is thick, add some salts as preservative.

The main ingredients for processing are sugar, salt, oil and grind spices. Such as cumin, cloves, coriander, cardamom, pepper and chillies. In Suri more or less 18 types of Morobba are prepared which have great demand in society. So regular annual income generation by the Morobba has great positive impact on the poverty mitigation or alleviation. Of the various types of Morobba the best tasty varieties are the Morobba of Am, Patol, Pepey, Satamuli, Akh and Amlaki. So, small-scale employment opportunity in the Morobba processing cottage industries for the inhabitant of Suri has created a good future prospect.

Cut into small pieces and soaked in water

↓

Drained out the water

↓

Peel the fruit pieces manually

↓

Remove the unwanted seeds

↓

If necessary grind the pulp to homogenize

↓

Boiled until the mixture is thickened

↓

Mixed the spices like cardamom etc. alongwith additives to give colour, flavour and taste. Pour into the lukewarm jars and sealed.

Fig. 1 : Flow Chart showing procurement of Morobba

Table 4

	Name of Morobba	*Botanical Name with Family*	*Parts Used*
1.	Ada (ginger)	*Zingiber officinale* Roxb. Zingiberaceae	Rhizome
2.	Kernel of Tal (palmyra palm)	*Borassus flabellifer* L. Arecaceae	Kernel
3.	Am (mango)	*Mangifera indica* L. Anacardiaceae	Fruit
4.	Thorh (Banana)	*Musa paradisiaca* L. Musaceae	Pseudostem
5.	Chaul-Kumrah (white gourd)	*Benincasa hispida* (Thunb.) Cucurbitaceae	Deseeded fruit pulp
6.	Kamranga (carambola)	*Averrhoa carambula* L. Oxalidaceae	Fruit
7.	Amlaki (embelic)	*Phyllanthus emblica* L. Euphorbiaceae	Fruit
8.	Akh (sugarcane)	*Saccharum officinarum* L. Poaceae	Stem

(Contd...)

(Table 4 – Contd...)

	Name of Morobba	Botanical Name with Family	Parts Used
9.	Bel (wood apple)	*Aegle marmelos* (L.) Corr. Rutaceae	Deseeded green or ripen fruit pulp
10.	Supari (betel-nut)	*Areca catechu* L. Arecaceae	Green fruit
11.	Satamuli (asparagus)	*Asparagus racemosus* Willd. Liliaceae	Tuberous root
12.	Pepey (papaya)	*Carica papaya* L. Caricaceae	Deseeded fruit pulp
13.	Patol (pointed gourd)	*Trichosanthes dioica* Roxb. Cucurbitaceae	Deseeded fruit
14.	Bahera (beleric)	*Terminalia bellirica* (Gaertn) Combretaceae	Fruit
15.	Khejur Methi (date palm)	*Phoenix sylvestris* L. Arecaceae	Fenugreek
16.	Haritaki (black myrobalan)	*Terminalia chebula* (Gaertn) Combretaceae	Fruit
17.	Anaros (Pine apple)	*Ananas comosus* Merr. Bromeliaceae	Fruit
18.	Kagji lebu (lime)	*Citrus aurantifolia* Swing. Rutaceae	Fruit

References

1. Douglas K. and Djendoel S. Discovery of Tarpenoid and phenolic sweeteners from plants, pure Appl chem, 2002 74(7), 1169-1179.
2. Inglett GE. A history of sweeteners- natural and synthetic, J. Toxicol Emeiron Health, 1976, 2(1), 207-214.
3. Sardesai VM and Waldshan TH, Natural and Synthetic intense sweeteners, J Nutr Biochem, 1991, 2(5), 236-244.
4. Kamble KD, Palm gur industry in India, Indian J Traditional Knowledge, 2003, 2(2) 137-147.
5. Sinku U, Ethnomedicinal use of rice beer (Deyang) among the tribe of Singhbum district of South Chotanagpur, In : Proc Natl Symp medicinal plants diversity in Chotanagpur Plateau and Human Welfare, Ranchi, Bihar, 1999, 5.
6. Kumar, V and Rao RR, Some interesting indigenous beverages among the tribals of Central India, Indian J Traditional Knowledge, 2007, 6(1), 141-143.

7. Aidoo KE, Nout MJR and Sarkar PK, Occurrence and function of yeasts in Asian indigenous fermented foods, FEMS Yeast Res, 2006, 6, 30.
8. Roy A, Moktan B and Sarkar PK, Traditional technology in preparing legume-based fermented foods of Orissa, IJTK, 2007, 6(1), 12–16.
9. Jain S.K., Glimpses of Indian Ethnobotany, (Oxford and IBH Publishing Co., New Delhi, India), 1981.
10. Jain S.K., Contributions to Ethnobotany of India, (Scientific Publishers, Jodhpur, India), 1991.
11. Jain S.K. and Rao R.R., A handbook of field and herbarium methods (Today and Tomorrow, Printers and Publishers, New Delhi), 1967, 33-58.
12. Efem SEE, Udoh KT and Iwara C, The antimicrobial spectrum of honey and its clinical significance. Infection, 1992, 20(4), 227-228.
13. Ghosh A, Apiphilic plants in agro-forestry. Natural Product Radiance, 2004, 3(3), 170.
14. Kandil A, El-Banby M, Abdel Wahed K, Abdel Gawwad M and Fayez M, Curative properties of true and floral and false non-floral noney on induced gastric ulcer. J. Drug Res (Cairo), 1987, 17(1-2), 103-105.
15. Aidoo KE, Nout MJR and Sarkar PK, Occurrence and function of yeasts in Asian indigenous fermented foods, FEMS Yeast Res, 2006, 6, 30.
16. Tamang JP, Sarkar PK and Hesseltine CW, Traditional fermented foods and beverages of Darjeeling and Sikkim-a review, J Sci Food Agric, 1988, 44, 375.
17. Chhetri RB and Gauchan DP, Traditional knowledge on fruit pulp processing of Lapsi in Kavrepalanchowk district of Nepal, IJTK, 2007, 6(1), 46-49.

3

Utilization of Natural Resources

3.1 Ethnobotanical Biocides of West Rarrh in West Bengal

Abstract

The study deals with the first-hand informations gathered during ethnobotanical surveys in South Bengal. Traditional uses by aborigines and rural folk for the treatment in plants, human and veterinary. The ethnobiocidal-lore of the tribes such as Bhumij, Chakma, Chero, Kharwar, Lodha, Mahali, Metch, Munda, Oraon, Rabha, Santal, Savar are presented in the table

Keywords : *Ethnopesticidal, West Rarrh, Decoction, Infusion.*

Introduction

A few decades of chemical development have led to severe damages to plants and animals through pollution. So, chemical pesticides are becoming major threats to living beings causing adverse side effects.

Keeping in mind, the study is presented on biocides the non-violent, cheaply available and healthy alternative used by tribes inhabited in West Rarrh region situated between the south side of the river Ganges and West side of the river Bhagirathi in West Bengal. This region is constituted by the districts of Murshidabad, Birbhum, Burdwan, Bankura, Purulia, Purba and Paschim Medinipur of W. Bengal. Its area is 27,500 Km^2.

Literature resume indicated that the region is under explored ethnobotanically. (Chattopadhyay and Maji 1975, Ghosh 2004).

Materials and Methods

The ethnobotanical surveys are carried out since 1995. The information is gathered from the tribal and rural medicinemen, farmers, repeated enquiries were made in different pockets of the region throughout the surveys. Plant specimens have collected, preserved and housed in the herbarium. Validity of data was confirmed by making queries among the villagers. Majority of them depend on indigenous herbal cures. External application is in the forms of powder, oil, paste, decoction and infusion etc.

Results and Discussion

The tribes and the farmers possess fairly good amount of indigenous knowledge about biocides against different diseases and pests. The data so far been achieved has verified several times by cross checking. This study enlightened on the popularity of our indigenous system of biocides which are still hidden among remote villagers. They await attention of phytochemists, pharmocologists and chemical engineers for further scientific research to divulge essential biocides for the well of living beings.

Table 1 : Systematic Enumeration of Plants Used as Remedies for the Outbreaks of the Pests and Diseases

Botanical Names and Family	*Vernacular Name*	*Parts Used*	*Pests/Disease*	*Preparation*
Adhatoda vasica Nees Acanthaceae	Basak	Leaf	Pest	Decoction
Aegle marmelos Corr. Rutaceae	Bel	Leaf	Pest	Decoction
Capsicum frutescens L. Solanaceae	Lanka	Fruit	Pest	Paste
Carica papaya L. *Caricaceae*	Pepey	Leaf	Spider, Larva	Decoction
Chrysanthenum coronarium L. Asteraceae	Chandramallika	Leaf	Ant, pest	Decoction
Cymbopogon citratus stap Poaceae	Lemon grass	Leaf	Pest, Stem rot, root rot, Burn spot	Oil + H_2O
Datura metel L. Solanaceae	Dhutra	Seed	Caterpillars	Powder + toddy
Jatropha curcas L. Euphorbiaceae	Bag-Bharenda	Leaf, Stem	Pest	Latex + Water
Dryopteris filix-mas L. Polypodiaceae	Fern	Plant	Powdery mildew of pea	Fresh extract
Lantana camara L. Verbenaceae	Bicha Phal/Kutush	Leaf, flower	Pest, late blight of potato	Decoction
Melia azadirachta L. Meliaceae	Neem	Leaf, fruit	Pest, diseases	Decoction
Michellia champaca L. Magnoliaceae	Champak	Flower	Pest	Fresh-juice
Moringa oleifera L. Moringaceae	Sajina	Leaf	Root rot	Decoction
Ocimum sanctum L. *Lamiaceae*	Kalo-tulsi	Leaf	Leaf scorch, leaf roll	Fresh juice
Opuntia dillenii Haw, Cactaceae	Phanimansha	Phylloclacde	Pest	Infusion
Ricinus communis L. Euphorbiaceae	Kerhi	Seed	Aphids, Larva	Oil + H_2O
Tagetes patula L. Asteraceae	Genda	Leaf, stem	Pest	Decoction
Vinca rosea L. Apocynaceae	Nayantara	Leaf	Flies	Fresh Juice
Vitex negundo L. Verbenaceae	Nicinda	Leaf	Pest	Decoction

3.2 Herbal Aromatic Ink in the Philetelic Stamp

Abstract

Humans are the aromaphilic. Aroma is the energy initiator and motivates sound health. In the present study the author has tried to focus the use of various vegetable scent in the philetelic stamp of the world.

Introduction

Great Britain is the pioneer (in 1840) for postal stamp service in the world history. Gradually it is widely spread in each country and we need postage stamp for use on mail articles and also in Valentine's day (14 Feb.). The stamp affixed on a letter indicates that the fees for carrying the letter to the addressee has already been paid to the postal department. Most of us buy stamps, use them and discarded them. However, a few people have the world's greatest hobby—The stamp collection. They find satisfaction in owning a variety of stamps of different scent, design etc. In fact, aromatic stamp collecting gradually become more popular and fascinating hobbies. Nearly 20 crore people around the world collect philetelic stamps. No wonder, it is called the "King of Hobbies". Now aromatic stamps are attractive work of miniature art and gives us immense joy and also may act as aromatherapy, induces sleep and relieve from all kinds of everyday stress. Keeping in mind the study is presented to aware everyone about various philetelic natural scent. The plants which are used to achieve scented smell in the philetelic stamps are given below in a tabular form.

Methods

During the philetelic collection these informations have been collected by author. The aromatic scent affixed in the backside of stamp by gum. Notes on the vegetable scents are presented.

Conclusion

The people should be convinced that the collection of philetelic stamp is beneficial for the livelihood and also for the

Valentine's day. These vegetable scented stamps are energetic and have no adverse side effect. It brings good news for the philetelist. Besides there are so many researches have done on aromatic stamps in Bhutan, South Korea, England etc. Maximum varieties of aromatic stamps are being available in South Korea. In near future vegetable scent may be widely used in any types of invitation card.

Table 2

Types of Scent	*Botanical Name and Family*	*Part Used*	*Name of Country with Year*
Rose	*Rosa centifolia* L. Rosaceae	Flower	Bhutan (Since 1973); South Korea (Since 2000)
Coffee	*Coffea arabica* L. Rubiaceae	Seeds	Brazil (Since 1999)
Lily	*Liliaceae*	Flower	South Korea (Since 2002)
Jasmine	*Jasminum auriculatum* Vahl Oleaceae	Flower	Australia (Since 2000)
Tea	*Camellia sinensis* L. Ternstroemiaceae	Leaf	Hongkong (Since 2000)
Chocolate	*Theobroma cacao* L. Sterculiaceae	Seed	Switzerland (Since 2001)
Tulip	*Sapathoda campanulata Liliaceae*	Flower	Netherland (Since 2002)
Dahlia	*Dahlia,* Asteraceae	Flower	Netherland
Orchid	*Vanilla planifolia* L. L. Orchidaceae	Flower	Nertherland
Eucalyptus	*Eucalyptus globulus* Myrtaceae	Leaf	
Apple	*Malus sylvestris* L. L. Rosaceae	Fruit	England
Anaros	*Ananas comosus* Merr. Bromeliaceae	Fruit	Russia (Since 2003)
Guava	*Psidium guajava* L. Myrtaceae	Fruit	Russia
Strawberry	*Fragaria vesica* Rosaceae	Fruit	Russia
Watermelon	*Citrullus vulgaris* Schr. Cucurbitaceae	Fruit	Russia
Sandal Wood	*Santalum album* L. Santalaceae	Wood	India (18 Dec. 2006)

3.3 Ethnobotanical Survey in West Rarrh (Murshidabad, Birbhum, Bankura, Purulia, Burdwan, Purba and Paschim Medinipur Districts) for Natural Health Care and Green Belt Movement

Abstract

Present scientific communication brings to knowledge the traditional methods of treating human diseases and disorders using plant-based drugs recorded from tribal and rural folks in West Rarrh region, West Bengal. A total of 48 plant species belonging to 31 families of angiosperms are employed by the inhabitants in the form of infusion, decoction, oil, paste, latex etc. either as a sole drug or in combination. The dose(s), duration and method of administration are given alongwith authentic botanical name, family, plant's part/form of recipe used and local plant names. The folk herbal formulations however require further modern laboratory testing.

Keywords *: Paschim Medinipur, Ethnomedicine, West Rarrh.*

Study Area

The hill tribes and aboriginals of West Rarrh are the Gonds, Kols, Mahali, Puraons Sabar (Kheria), Lodha, Munda, Santal, Oraon, Bhumij, Mech, Bedia etc. from the immemorial time. The West Rarrh of W. Bengal mainly constituted the districts of Murshidabad, Burdwan, Birbhum, Bankura, Purulia and Midnapore. It is the extended part of Chhotanagpur plateau. Here the forests are distributed roughly in an isosceles triangle with the base running north and south, from the tip of Birbhum district to the southern part of Midnapore district. Forest lie scattered in small patches between latitude 21° 75′ to 24° 33′N and longitudes 85° 70′ to 87° 80′E. Its area is 27,500 Km^2. Here the hills are relict type. The remarkable hills are Beharinath and Sushunia lie among Bankura district. The forests are in the laterite soil through which main rivers like Ajay, Maurakshi, Damodar, Shilabati etc. run roughly west to east fall into Hoogly while the Subarnarekha flows independently and fall into the Bay of Bengal. In West Rarrh three types of soil (alluvial, red and laterite) are present.

Basically dominance of hot and humid climate alogwith a short duration of winter (December to January). Temperature reaches its maximum (39.45°C in average) in the month of May and falls in the month of January (12.57°C). South west monsoon is the chief source of rains. Rainfall continues from the June to September. Major crops of this region are rice, maize, groundnut, potato etc. Here the dominant trees in the forest are *Shorea robusta, Madhuca indica, Terminalia chebula, Terminalia bellirica* etc. The denuded or blank areas have been afforested chiefly by *Eucalyptus globolus, Tectona grandis, Acacia auriculiformis* etc.

The total population of West Rarrh of West Bengal is 2,19,67,823. Of which, population of schedule tribes (ST) are 19,40,842 (Census-1991). Bhumij, Lodhas, Kherias, Mundas, Mahalis, Santals generally build small huts. Catching fish, crabs etc. by bamboo traps, nets, and palm fibers and creepers like *Ichnocarpus frutescens* and also by different poisonous plants like *Euphorbiaantiquorum* etc. Besides catching of tortoise, iguana, rat-snake, bat, squirrel, larva of red ants, cocoons is the general practices of the tribals. Tribals have traditional craft like bamboo based combs, basket, weaving of mats and brooms of different plants.

Lodha, Sabar and Munda etc. have their some own traditional peculiarities such as the mother is given some Kurthi water (*Dolichos biflorus*) just after delivery followed by mother alongwith the new born baby are bathed with turmeric water (*Curcuma longa*) on the 9th day of delivery.

Introduction

Plants have been used as a source of medicine for living beings from ancient times. According to an estimate of WHO, approximately 80% of the people in developing countries rely chiefly on traditional medicines for primary healthcare. Ethno medicinal survey, help mankind to search and develop new cures to treat various ailments. The inhabitants of the study area have rich heritage particularly related to plant utility and the literature survey shows that the region was almost untapped from this point of view (Jain and De 1964; Kar 1999; Ghosh

2002, 2003). The pioneer workers (Cox 1994; Jain 1963, 1989) contributing a lot in the field of ethnobotanical research. The present communication focussed some more plant species from this region.

Materials and Methods

Ethnobotanical field explorations were carried out during the years 2001-2003 in between the age group of 50-70. Information of folk-medicinal use of plants was obtained through oral interviews enduring local plant name, parts used, other ingredients added (if any), method of preparation and mode of administration etc. for each species. Plant specimens were collected from the study area, authenticated and kept in the Herbarium of the institute. The ethno-medical information is presented in tabular form (Table 3).

Table 3 : Ethnomedicinally Important Plants of West Rarrh

Ailments	*Local Name*	*Botanical Name and Family*	*Parts Used*	*Recipe*	*Administration*
Tumour	Sasha	*Cucumis sativus L. (Ghosh 112)* (Cucurbitaceae)	Fruit	One fresh fruit (100 gm)	Consumed raw once daily to prevent cancer.
	Bilati Begun	*Lycopersicum esculemum* Mill. (Ghosh 193) (Solanaceae)	Fruit	Fruit	Consumed raw.
Snake's bite (Boas)	Kantal	*Artocarpus heterophyllus* Lamk. (Ghosh 39) (Moraceae)	Peduncle	Juice	Fed 1 cup juice thrice daily immediately after bite. Till complete cure in achieved.
Snake bite	Iswarnul	*Aristolochia indica L.* (Ghosh 38) (Aristolochiaceae)	Bark, root	Juice	Fed to the human and cows 1-2 cup juice twice daily till cure.
Food poison	Arimed	*Acacia leucophloea (Rosb.) Willd* (Ghosh 326) (Mimosaceae)	Bark, latex	Juice	Fed 1 cup immediately.
Blood vomitting	Berela	*Sida cordifolia* L. (Ghosh 274) (Malvaceae)	Root, leaf	Crushed and made into paste	Fed 1 cup immediately.
Accumulation of fat	Nishinda	*Vitex negundo* L. (Ghosh 319) (Verbenaceae)	Leaf	Juice	One teaspoonful fed daily for 45 days alongwith few drops of lemon (lime-kagji) juice.
Accumulation of fat	Mangustan	*Garcinia mangostana* L. (Ghosh 327) (Guttiferae)	Leaf, husk	Juice	One tea spoonful fed daily for 30 days.
Pain in teeth (toothache)	Gorap-Begun	*Solanum virginianum* L. (Ghosh 279) (Solanaceae)	Root	Fresh root	Grind the root by the affected teeth.

(Contd...)

(Table 3 – Contd...)

Ailments	Local Name	Botanical Name and Family	Parts Used	Recipe	Administration
Anti-fertility	Nagdona	*Artimisia vulgaris L.* (Ghosh 328) (Asteraceae)	Leaf, root	Crushed and made into 10g. tablet	10 tablets in each cycle claimed to be contraceptive.
Impotence	Shialkanata	*Argemone mexicana* L. (Ghosh 37) (Papaveraceae)	Seed, plant latex	Crushed seeds, with its latex	5 g. paste taken daily for 30 days to cure.
Blood dysentery/ Diarrhoea/	Ramdatan	*Smilax macrophylla* Roxb. (Ghosh 275) (Liliaceae)	Root	Juice	Drunk ½ cup juice twice daily till complete cure is achieved.
Night Wetting	Ulatkambal	*Abroma augusta* L. (Ghosh 2) (Sterculiaceae)	Root	Juice	Drunk ½ cup juice once daily till complete cure is achieved.
Wasp bite	Baichi	*Flacourtia indica* (Burm f.) Merr. (Ghosh 153) (Flacourtiaceae)	Stem, bark	Fresh bark	Apply 10g. paste on the wound
Alopecia/Boils Wounds	Karanj	*Caesalpinia crista* L. (Ghosh 63) (Caesalpiniaceae)	Seed	Oil extracted from seeds	Hair, boils and wounds smeared with oil till complete cure is achieved.
Diabetes mellitus	Karanj	*Caesalpinia crista* L (Ghosh 63) (Caesalpiniaceae)	Leaf	Crushed 10 leaves and made into paste	Fed to the patient once daily for 7 days.
Dandruff/ Premature hair greying	Sikaki	*Acaccia concinna* DC. (Ghosh 8) (Leguminosae)	Leaf, seed	Juice	Regular external applications administered.
Mis-carriage (abortion)	(*i*) Anantamul (*ii*) Daruchini	*Hemidesmus indicus* R. Br. (Ghosh 165) (Asclepiadaceae) *Cinnamomum zeylanica* Breyn. (Ghosh 88) (Lauraceae)	Root Bark	2-2 gm roots of anantamul and 2 gm of daruchini boiled in a glass of cow's milk.	Administered orally to the patient once a day for 7 days.

(Contd...)

(Table 3 – Contd...)

Ailments	Local Name	Botanical Name and Family	Parts Used	Recipe	Administration
Acne	Ayapan	*Eupatorium ayapana* Vent. BP. (Ghosh 139) (Asteraceae)	Leaf	Juice	Externally apply on the face.
Alopecia	Datura	*Datura metel* L. (Ghosh 121) (Solanaceae)	Leaf	Juice	Massage the juice on head for 30 minutes.
Acne/Alopecia	(*i*) White Sarisha	*Brassica campestris* L. (Ghosh 57) (Brassicaceae)	Seed	Both seeds (1:1 ratio) crushed and made into paste	Externally applied on head in Alopecia and at face for Acne (pimple).
	(*ii*) Til	*Sesamum indicum* DC. (Ghosh 270) (Pedaliaceae)	Seed		
Miliaria rubra (Miliary)	Anantamul	*Hemidesmus indicus* R.Br. (Ghosh 165) (Asclepiadaceae)	Root	Juice	Rubbed on the body.
Kidney stone	Mashkalai	*Vigna mungo* (L.) Hepper. (Ghosh 229) (Papilionaceae)	Cotyleden	Infusion	A cup of infusion drunk at morning till complete cure is achieved.
Food poisoning in cows	Iswarmul	*Aristolochia indica* L. (Ghosh 38) (Aristolochiaceae)	Bark, root	Juice	Fed to the cows.
Diarrhoea in cows	Swarnalata	*Cuscuta reflexa* Roxb (Ghosh 117) (Cuscutaceae)	Stem	Juice	Fed to the cows thrice daily till cure.
Cuts and wounds	Bherenda	*Jatropha curcas* L (Ghosh 180) (Euphorbiaceae)	Latex	Fresh Latex	Latex smeared on the wound
Cuts and wounds	Kamini	*Murraya paniculata* Jack (L.) (Ghosh 211) (Rutaceae)	Leaf	Powder	Apply powder to check bleeding.

(Contd...)

(Table 3 – Contd...)

Ailments	*Local Name*	*Botanical Name and Family*	*Parts Used*	*Recipe*	*Administration*
Weak nerves of leg	Pan	*Piper betle* L. (Ghosh 238) (Piperaceae)	Leaf	Green leaves	Fed one raw leaf daily alongwith honey for 30 days.
Louse infestation	Boch	*Acorus calamus* L. (Ghosh 12) (Araceae)	Rhizome	Infusion	Applied infusion on affected parts.
Diabetes mellitus	Currypata	*Murraya koenigii* (L.) Spreng. (Ghosh 210) (Rutaceae)	Leaf	Fresh leaves	Fed 10 leaflets once daily before lunch.
Infertility	Bon-dhenros	*Malachra capitata* L. (Ghosh 195) (Malvaceae)	Fruit	Fresh fruit	Fed to the patient 5 raw fruits daily during menstrual period for 3 months.
Asthma	Dayalu flower	*Aerva lanata* L. Schult (Ghosh 17) (Amaranthaceae)	Flower with leaf	Juice	Drunk 5 ml juice with few drops of honey for one month.
Infertility	Swet-lajjabati	*Mimosa pudica* L. (Ghosh 203) (Mimosaceae)	Root	Juice	Drunk one tea spoonful juice alongwith a pepper (*P. nigrum*) for 20 days.
	Swet-aparajita	*Clitoria ternatea* L. (Ghosh 98) (Caesalpineae)	Root	Juice	Do
Low blood-pressure	Bon-kalmi	*Ipomoea paniculata* R. Br. (Ghosh 179) (Convolvulaceae)	Leaf	Juice	Drunk ½ cup juice once daily for 15 days.
Enlargemnt of Liver/Dim sighted	Bon-charal	*Desmodium gyrans* DC. (Ghosh 126) (Fabaceae)	Leaf	Juice	Drunk 2 spoonful juice daily.

(Contd...)

(Table 3 – Contd...)

Ailments	Local Name	Botanical Name and Family	Parts Used	Recipe	Administration
Small pox	Swet Kantikari	*Solanum virginianum* L (Ghosh 279) (Solanaceae)	Aerial part	Crushed and made into paste	2 dry tablets consumed daily for 7 days as an antidote both in human and cow.
Hydrophobia	(*i*) Bans	*Bambusa vulgaris* Schrad. (Ghosh 330) (Poaceae)	Root	Crushed in (1:1) ratio.	Administered orally (50g.) and externally applied on the wound made by dog bite as an antidote.
	(*ii*) Ankar	*Alangium salviifolium* (L.f.) Wang. (Ghosh 19) (Alangiaceae)	Root		
Snake bite	Barachadar	*Rauvolfia canescens* L. (Ghosh 225) (Apocynaceae)	Root	Juice	Drunk 10 ml juice and also apply the juice on the wound.
Diabetes mellitus	Barachadar	*Rauvolfia canescens L.* (Ghosh 225) (Apocynaceae)	Root	Juice	Fed to patient alongwith *Terminalia arjuna* bark.
Diabetes mellitus	Gudmar, Meshsringi	*Gymnema sylvestre* R. Br. (Ghosh 161) (Asclepiadaceae)	Leaf, fruit	Juice	Drunk 5 ml juice once daily for 30 days before lunch.
Constipation	Golmorich	*Piper nigrum* L. (Ghosh 240) (Piperaceae)	Fruit	Powder	Powder (5g.) mixed in a cup of lukewarm water drunk at night.
Flatulence	Kul	*Ziziphus mauritiana* Lamk. (Ghosh 324) (Rhamnaceae)	Leaf	Paste	Paste rubbed on abdomen.
High Bilirubin (Billiousness)	Bhui Amla	*Phyllanthus niruri auct. pL.* (Ghosh 237) (Euphorbiaceae)	Whole plant	Juice	Drunk 5 ml. juice once daily for 10 days before lunch.

(Contd...)

(Table 3 – Contd...)

Ailments	*Local Name*	*Botanical Name and Family*	*Parts Used*	*Recipe*	*Administration*
Jaundice	Chichinga	*Trichosanthes anguina* L. (Ghosh 303) (Cucurbitaceae)	Leaf, seed	Juice	Drunk 5 ml juice once daily for 7 days.
Bedsore	Nishinda	*Vitex negundo* L. (Ghosh 319) (Verbenaceae)	Leaf	Paste	Smear in affected region.
Alopecia	(*i*) Ghrita-kumari (*ii*) Methi	*Aloe vera* L. (Ghosh 24) (Liliaceae) *Trigonella foenum graecum* L. (Ghosh 331) (Fabaceae)	Intact leaf juice Seed	Methi seeds germinated in the leaf juice of *A. vera*	The decoction of germinated seeds alongwith coconut oil is applied externally.
Burn, Rough skin	Ghrita-kumari	*Aloe vera* L. (Ghosh 24) (Liliaceae)	Fresh leaf juice	Juice	Smear in skin.
Epilepsy	Shet Karabi	*Nerium indicum* Mill. (Ghosh 215) (Apocynaceae)	Root	Juice	Drunk 5 ml juice once daily for 15 days.

Results and Discussion

Locally available plants are used by the people as their household remedies. The data has been accrued from the tribal and rural people of the 7 districts which still find place their traditional therapy. However, isolation of active principles, phytochemical and pharmacological investigations are desired to validate the claims of the traditional healers. This may provide new sources of herbal drugs. The formulation of these effective phyto-medicines should be encouraged for their sustainable uses. Statistically, information for treating a particular ailment from different informants certainly reflects the accuracy and authenticity of the folk drugs employed.

The villages of the region are rich in ethno-medicinal knowledge owing to their close affinity with the surrounding plant cover. They obtain a variety of plant products from wild plants to fulfill their own needs as they are economically weaker sections of the society. In the tribal areas the rules and regulations by which the tribal people have been traditionally governed are now being gradually abolished by the young literate generations. Another crucial factor responsible for such change is the migration of youth from tribal areas to urban areas. This gap is further widened the adoption of modern medicine. Therefore, the importance of recording indigenous knowledge base related technology as described here become essential in view of rapid socioeconomic and cultural changes and for high tech low cost solution. Religious and cultural faith, poor economy and lack of modern medical facilities in villages of the study area seems to be the cause of utilisation of these plants. While conducting the survey the inhabitant revealed that most of the people were dependent on plants and they also preferred it, although the preparing methods are known only to local faith healers. Due to rapid increase in human and consequent increased population biotic interference some species are dwindling from their natural habitats. It is, therefore, imperative that green medicines of the aborigines which are still in vogue should be documented for obvious reasons.

3.4 Traditional House-hold Things Made by the Potters of West-Rarrh

Abstract

The indigenous technical knowledge (ITK) of the potters has been focused which are gradually being abolishing due to industrial revolution. Potters generally process those house-hold things which have traditional value of income generation.

Keywords : Indigenous technical knowledge, Potters, Banak clay.

Introduction

From ancient time a man is known by his profession. At that time there was no service. In course of time in the society there evolved so many professional men due to division of labour such as oil-man, milkman, fisherman, washerman, boat-man, blacksmith, farmer, carpenter, weaver, barber, goldsmith, cobbler, potter etc which are still existing. Of them potters are in miserable situation as the clay made house-hold utensils (earthen-wares) are replaced by iron, steel, bell-metal, copper, silver, brass, fibre, tin, glass-ware, plastic etc. and at the same time quality as well as texture and temper of the soil is gradually diminishing due to indiscriminate use of chemical fertilizer in the soil from 1960's. Fifty years ago the longevity of clay-walls are of near about 100-150 years. But today it lasts for 50-90 years. As a result potters and mud-house makers are facing the serious problems to survive. Till now different kinds of clay-pots are indispensable for traditional rituals and to prepare parched rice, fried rice, cheese, butter milk, solid thickened milk, whey, beers, beverages, cold drinks, etc due to its percolating properties which are totally absent in different metal-pots, plastic pots, fibre pots, glass wares etc.

Materials and Methods

Generally sand mixed clay soil are collected by the potters from the bank of big tanks at 1 meter depth at the advent of summer or during the winter months and preserved it for use round the year. After giving the desired shape of things by potter's wheel they roasted it in the thatched fire oven of potter's kiln or pottery (*i.e.* a large furnace for calcining). The red showy Banak clay dye is obtained from 1–2.5 m depth in the crop fields which is used in earthen pitcher, cooking pots, tiles, walls etc. Usually 500 kg Bank clay yields 50 kg dye.

Results and Discussion

The age of the clays in West-Rarrh is approximately 65 million years (Ghosh 2004) and the potters engaged in this profession for near about thousand years. Here the colour of the clay varies from white to brown, pink or black. Potters sometimes exported the Banak clay dyes in the other states of India. The dye gives protection against salinity to earthen pots and other things and at the same time increase the beauty. The cost of earthen wares varies depending on its size and colour. Generally the cost of a pitcher is Rs. 6–12, frying pan is Rs. 30–35, tub is Rs. 35–40, large basin or reservoir for soaking the boiled paddy for overnight in water is Rs. 60–100 etc. Poor farmers use the small basin in their cow-shed for thoroughly wetting the rice dust and fodder.

Kinds of Utensils alongwith their Vernacular Names of West-Rarrh are mentioned below :

Pitcher (kalsi), jug (kujo), kettle, tub (gamla), pan (karah), ewer (garu), glass, tea-cup (khuri), plate (thala), doll (putul), lamp (pradip), cup (bati), jar (jala), lid (dhakna), pot (harhi), lampstand (pilsuj), flower-vase (fuldani), frying pan (khola), foolish-vessel (boka-varh), water-vessel (jhari), water-pot (ghot), round earthen pot (malsa), earthen lid (sora), incense pot (dhunachi), grinder (janta).

Of them kettle, pan, pot, frying pan, plate etc. are used in cooking industry and pitcher, jug, tub, ewer, glass, jar etc. are used to keep the drinking water in cool condition during summer month. Lamp, lamp-stand, flower-vase, water-pot, round earthen pot, earthen pot, earthen lid, incense pot, dolls etc. are popularly used in different rituals. Earthen pots have a great demand for fermenting rice beer; and to prepare the rice-cake (garh-garhey pitha) water vessels are indispensable (Roy *et al.* 2007). Earthern pots are the best container to keep the molasses in good condition.

3.5 Natural Dye Making Process Alongwith its Dye Yielding Plants of West Rarrh

Abstract

Natural dye is an integral part of human health care system compared to synthetic dyes as they have no adverse side effects and toxicity. The present study is an attempt to investigate the dye yielding plants alongwith their vernacular names, how different part(s) are used in dye procurement etc. 60 plant species belonging to 35 families of ethnodyeing interest are recorded after critical screening.

Keywords : *Dye yielding plants, West Rarrh, Mordants.*

Introduction

From ancient time people advocates the use of plants as dye resource. Dye obtained from plant origin occupy important position in modern life. Data on the plant dye uses have been systematically gathered and compiled by many workers (Ghosh 2009, Gokhale *et. al.*, 2004, Gaur 2008). History reveals that Chinese have recorded the use of dye even before 2600 B.C. The most common dyes are extracting from leaves, stems, barks, roots, fruits, flowers and seeds. Degradable eco-friendly dyes are one of the most important uses of plants, as it relates with cultural practices, rituals, arts and crafts etc.

West Rarrh is located in the south part of West Bengal in between latitudes 21°75′ to 24°33′ N and longitudes 85°70′ to 87°80′ E, and acquires 27,000 sq km geographical area. The tract covers the Civil Districts of Purba and Paschim Medinipur, Bankura, Purulia, Burdwan, Birbhum and Murshidabad. The population of this region is heterogeneous, associated with so many tribal communities like Bedia, Bhumij, Birhor, Jatorh, Lodha, Mahali, Mahato (Kurmi), Metch, Munda, Oraon, Santal, Savar (Kheria) etc. The main occupation of the people is agriculture, livestock farming, preying, wood based profession, including yielding of natural dyes. Tribal communities are well acquainted with various herbal dyes which are remained unveiled. Considering the importance of traditional knowledge and future prospectus of eco-friendly dyes the present study is an extensive effort to record some information about dye procurement process from dye yielding plants of which some are gradually being abolished.

Materials and Methods

An extensive field survey was conducted in the rural and tribal pockets of West Rarrh since 1995. The detailed information on dye yielding plants alongwith dye procurement process was recorded through personal interviews. The collected plant specimens have been authenticated by a taxonomist (Dr. Manindranath Sanyal, Ex-Prof of Bishnupur Ramananda College). Plant species used by the tribals are mentioned in Table with their botanical and vernacular names, family and their part(s) used as dye.

Techniques of Extraction of Dyes

(*a*) To extract dye from rhizome, root, stem or bark, the raw material is cut into small pieces, soaked in water for 2–3 days and made into paste. After squeezing and filtration, the whole extract is boiled to achieve desirable concentration.

(*b*) For fruit and rinds the material is squeezed and the juice is added with required amount of water. This solution is kept in iron or earthen pots for 2–3 days which are act as a mordant.

(*c*) The plants and leaves used for dye are crushed and dissolved in water for 12–24 hrs followed by gentle heating to achieve desirable concentration.

The dye colour varied depending on the type of mordants. Some vegetable dyes are used as mordants (Nishidak and Kabayashi 1992). Light solution of organic manure, cow urine or cow dung, whey, curd water, wood ash, lime water, lemon juice, rock salt are common mordants used by the tribals.

By adopting such measures vegetable dye resources are very helpful in the ecofriendly development of concerned industries (such as chromotherapy depends on natural dyes) and thereby combat against pollution. Recently red soil of West Rarrh rich in Fe, Al or Cu compounds together with plant dyes *i.e., Acacia catechu, Semecarpus anacardium* (bhelai or marking nut) etc. are used by the tribals in wall painting and in pottery (Ghosh 2009, Mathpal 1995). Besides black ink is prepared by the tribal student from *Eclipta alba, Semecarpus anacardium* etc. For ink making dye yielding part is gently heated with water followed with filtration and the solution is kept in earthen pots and added some alum, lac etc. as mordant.

Results and Discussion

By mid 1800, Chemists began to producing synthetic substitutes for herbal dye but at present due to ban on production of some of the synthetic dyes due to their harmful problem the demand of natural dye is gradually increasing in textile industry, pottery industry, food and beverage industry etc. The creation of a bond between the colouring matter and fibre is called mordanting *i.e.* a pre-dyeing process that makes the fibre receptive to dye. Mordant is a chemical that when cooked with fibres attaches itself to the fibre molecules. Generally a dye molecule attaches itself to the mordant. Herbal dye are susceptible to mordant which are metallic salts of Al, Fe, Cu and others for ensuring the reasonable fastness of the colour to sunlight and also washing. The vessel that is used for dyeing itself is serving as a mordant. Generally dye yielders use copper, tin vessels to brighten the colour and iron pan to dull the colour. To achieve basic original colour earthen or stainless steel pots are desirable.

Majority of dye resource belong to dicot and are of common occurrence. Dyes are produced from various parts of the plant *i.e.* leaf, stem, bark, root, rhizome, flower, fruit, seed, resin etc. Generally chlorophyll, the source of green colour is easily extracted with the help of solvents like alcohol or acetone (Arnon 1949). As most of the natural dyes are feeble. So, their fastness or longevity depends on the use of mordants.

There is a global demand for plant dyes as it is biodegradable. As the methods of collection and extraction of dyes (*i.e.* procuring process) are still crude and traditional so further research is required to strengthen the dye yielding process, and the whole process will be delightful if it is incorporated in work education project as a self employment tool for the student.

Table 4 : Dye Yielding Plants of West Rarrh

Sl. No.	*Botanical Name*	*Vernacular Name*	*Family*	*Parts Used*	*Dye Procured*
1.	*Abrus precatorious L.*	Kunch	Fabaceae	Seed	Black
2.	*Acacia catechu Willd.*	Khair	Mimosaceae	Wood	Dark-brown
3.	*A. nilotica Willd. Ex Del.*	Babla	–do–	Rind/ gum	Black
4.	*Achyranthes aspera L.*	Apang	Amaranthaceae	Whole plant	Black-brown
5.	*Adhatoda zeylanica* Medic.	Basak	Acanthaceae	Leaf	Yellow-green
6.	*Aegle marmelos (L.) Corr.*	Bel	Rutacene	Bark/ fruit	Yellow
7.	*Anacardium occidentale L.*	Kaju badam	Anacardiaceae	Pericarp	Light red
8.	*Annona squamosa L.*	Ata	Annonaceae	Fruit	Yellow
9.	*Annona reticulata L.*	Nona	–do–	–do–	Bluish-black
10.	*Artocarpus heterophyllus Lamk.*	Kathal	Moraceae	Fruit/ wood	Yellow
11.	*A. lakoocha Roxb.*	Madar	–do–	–do–	–do–
12.	*Averrhoa carambula L.*	Kamranga	Oxalidaceae	Fruit	Yellow-brown
13.	*Bauhinia purpurea L.*	Raktakanchan	Caesalpiniaceae	Bark	Purple
14.	*B. variegata L.*	Kanchan	–do–	Flower	–do–
15.	*Beta vulgaris L.*	Beet	Chenopodiaceae	Root	Red
16.	*Bixa orellana L.*	Lotkon	Bixaceae	Pulp (aril)	Orange Yellow

(Contd...)

(Table 4 – Contd...)

Sl. No.	Botanical Name	Vernacular Name	Family	Parts Used	Dye Procured
17.	*Bougainvillea glabra* Choisy	Baganbilas	Nyctaginaceae	Flower	Yellow
18.	*Butea monosperma (Lamk.) Taub*	Palash	Fabaceae	–do–	Yellow-orange
19.	*B. superba Roxb.*	Lata palash	–do–	Root	Orange
20.	*Carthamus tinctorius L.*	Kusum	Asteraceae	Flower	Red
21.	*Cassia fistula L.*	Sondal	Caesalpiniaceae	Bark/ fruits	Brown
22.	*C. tora L.*	Chakunda	–do–	Seed	Blue
23.	*Casuarina equisetifolia Forst.*	Jhau	Casuarinaceae	Bark	Light red
24.	*Cinnamomum tamala (Buch-Ham.)*	Tejpata	Lauraceae	Leaf	Brown
25.	*Commelina benghahalensis L.*	Kanshira	Commelinaceae	Flower	Blue
26.	*Curcuma aromatica Salisb.*	Ban halud	Zingiberaceae	Rhizome	Yellow
27.	*C. longa L.*	Halud	–do–	–do–	–do–
28.	*Daucas carota L.*	Gajor	Apiaceae	Root	–do–
29.	*Eclipta alba L.*	Keshute	Asteraceae	Leaf	Black
30.	*Grewia asiatica L.*	Phalsa	Tiliaceae	Fruit	Yellow-orange
31.	*Hibiscus rosa sinensis L.*	Jaba	Malvaceae	Leaf	Red
32.	*Impatiens balsamina L.*	Dopati	Balsaminaceae	Flower	Red
33.	*Indigofera tinctoria L.*	Nil	Fabaceae	Leaf	Blue
34.	*Lagerstroemia parviflora Roxb.*	Shida	Lythraceae	Bark	Black
35.	*Lannea coromandelica (Houth) Merr.*	Jial	Anacardiaceae	–do–	Yellow-brown
36.	*Lawsonia inermis L.*	Mehndi	Lythraceae	Leaf	Yellow-orange
37.	*Madhuca indica Gmelin*	Mahua	Sapotaceae	Bark	Reddish yellow

(Contd...)

(Table 4 – Contd...)

Sl. No.	Botanical Name	Vernacular Name	Family	Parts Used	Dye Procured
38.	*Mangifera indica L.*	Am	Anacardiaceae	Bark/ Leaf	Yellow
39.	*Mimusops elengi L.*	Bokul	Sapotaceae	Bark	Brown
40.	*Mirabilis jalapa L.*	Sandhyamoni	Nyctaginaceae	Flower	Pink-red
41.	*Musa paradisiaca L.*	Kanchkala	Musaceae	Pseudo stem	Black
42.	*Nyctanthes arbor-tristis L.*	Sheuli	Oleaceae	Flower	Yellow-orange
43.	*Nymphaea alba L.*	Shaluk	Nymphaeaceae	Rhizome	Blue
44.	*Phyllanthus emblica L.*	Amlaki	Euphorbiaceae	Fruit	Blue-black
45.	*Psidium guajava L.*	Peyara	Myrtaceae	–do–	Black-brown
46.	*Pterocarpus marsupium Roxb.*	Piasal	Fabaceae	Bark	Brow-nish red
47.	*Punica granatum L.*	Dalim	Punicaceae	Fruit rind	Yellow-red
48.	*Rubia cordifolia L.*	Manjistha	Rubiaceae	Stem root	Red-brown
49.	*R. tinctoria L.*	Madder	–do–	Root	Red
50.	*Semecarpus anacardium L.f.*	Bhelai	Ancardiaceae	Fruit	Black
51.	*Syzygium cumini (L.) Skeels*	Jam	Myrtaceae	–do–	Black/ purple
52.	*Tagetes erecta L.*	Genda	Asteraceae	Flower	Yellow
53.	*T. patula L.*	–do–	–do–	–do–	Brown
54.	*Tamarindus indica L.*	Tentul	Caesalpiniaceae	Leaf	Reddish yellow
55.	*Tectona grandis L.f.*	Sagoon	Verbenaceae	Bark	Reddish
56.	*Terminalia arjuna Roxb.*	Arjun	Combretaceae	–do–	Light brown
57.	*T. bellirica (Gaertn.) Roxb.*	Bahera	–do–	Fruit	Blue
58.	*T. chebula Retz.*	Haritaki	–do–	–do–	Yellow
59.	*Woodifordia fruticosa (L.) Kurz.*	Dhatri phul	Lythraceae	Flower	Red
60.	*Ziziphus jujuba (L.) Lamk.*	Kul	Rhamnaceae	Fruit	Reddish pink

3.6 Sustainable Dolls from Ant-Hill

Abstract

Potential value of easily available natural Ant-hills are used by us in making Jau-dolls have been discussed in this article for further improvement and self-employment. Without ant-hill soil Jau-dolls can not be created, though Jau-dolls are valuable for ornamenting the drawing room.

Keywords : Anti-hill, West Bengal, Jau-doll, Lac.

Introduction

Many species of animals eat dirt as medicine to rectify mineral deficiencies in their diet. Chimpanzees, giraffes, elephants and rhinoceroses eat regular mouthfuls of clay-rich termite, mound soil. Ant-hill is an effective binding agent as its chemical structure allows other chemicals to bond with it. Besides ant-hill soil is an effective deactivator of toxins in the gouty organs. Ant-hill is an excellent materials made by termites in the waste places which are being used for Jau-dolls. The ant larvae are used in prey for fish and as a consequence indirectly save the woods, textiles, furnitures, books etc.

Materials and Methods

At first the collected ant-hills are grounded into dust. The dusts are made into chyme with the help of demineralised water (preferably rain water). The chymes are cut into desirable pieces and give the various shapes of animals, men and idols by using the fingers. These raw dolls are then kept in sunlight for 2–3 days followed by roasting on cow dung cake fuel oven. In the next phase lacs are melted by iron-pan over the wood fire. The dried dolls are varnished by melted lac sticks. At the end the dolls are coloured by desirable vegetable dye mixed in lac. The dolls size are generally ranges in between 2–15 inches and their cost varies from Rs. 10–500.

Results and Discussion

The whole process is executed well during winter. We are

the leading innovator in West Bengal for the production of Jau dolls and thereby proper utilization of ant-hills can takes place which are very effective for our daily life. Potters can earn money by self-employment. Lac is generally grown on host trees of kusum (*Schleichera oleosa* Oken), Palash (*Butea monosperma* Taub) and Kul (*Zizyphus jujuba* Lamk) found abundantly in the forest of Purulia, Bankura and Paschim Medinipur district. People residing inside the forest or in the fringe areas are depending completely for their livelihood on lac production (Siddiqui 2004).

In secondary schools the students can be trained through workshop on work education to develop manpower for Jau dolls production by adopting feedback system. By adopting it as career, mass migration of youth from interior villages to towns can be checked. At the same time deforested natural forest where large number of wild sapling and trees of lac host trees are available are required to be conserved for fruitful future employment opportunities for coming generation. Ant-hill is an important ingredient as household balm against arthritis. Due to its wonderful characteristics has a wide range of applications as balm.

3.7 Tea Plants Used as Veterinary Medicine in Farmers Daily Life

Abstract

Though tea is the most widely used beverage in the world still so, many ailments of buffaloes, cows, sheeps, horses, goats and dogs can be cured by tea plants. In the present study an attempt was made to unveil the preventive properties of tea.

Keywords : *Tea, Green Tea, Black Tea, White Tea, Beverage.*

Introduction

The modern term 'Tea' derives from early Chinese dialect word cha. Though from 2737 BC (the Chinese Emperor, Shen Nung time) tea was renowned for its beverage property. Now it is widely used for its medicinal properties. Tea botanically known as *Thea sinensis* Linn., is an evergreen plant of the Theaceae family. Tea varieties are currently considered as promising herbal medicine for the future (Cao 1997, Deng *et. al.*, 1998, Thelle 1995).

Extensive research for the last 17 years seems to prove that tea is a health drink for domestic animals (Sharma, 2000). The ability of tea to lower serum glucose levels thereby acting as anti-ageing and antidiabetic (Devi *et. al.*, 2004), tea may reduce the intestinal absorption of glucose (Kreydiyyeh *et. al.*, 1994) and have a strong sugar lowering action (Karawya *et. al.*, 1984). Preventive effect of green tea consumption in heart disease (Thelle, 1995) and also reduce the risk of high blood cholesterol alongwith high blood pressure (Stensvold, 1992). Providing tea polyphenols in the drinking water of animals increases the enzyne activity of liver (Khan *et. al.*, 1992) to aids digestion and detoxification.

Table 5

Ailments	*How Medicine is Prepared*	*How Used*
Swelling throat due to cold and pneumonia	Tea-dust along with a pinch rock salt.	Lukewarm Tea bags locally applied externally twice daily for 3–4 days.
Milk production	Tea dust alongwith a pinch of urea in lukewarm water claimed to enhance milk production in cows.	
Sting bite		Used tea bags on the wound to bring down the swelling and pain.
Asthma	Tea-the healthy drinks are the instant reliver	
Flatulence	Crushed 10 seeds of pepper alongwith 2 spoon of tea-dust and a pinch of rock salt.	Fed the mixture alongwith 100 gm molasses twice daily to domestic animals.
Diarrhoea	Ingestion of 3 tea leave alongwith 3 leaves of *Piper betle L.*	Twice daily to check.

(Contd...)

(Table 5 – Contd...)

Ailments	*How Medicine is Prepared*	*How Used*
Cough/cold	Fed the drink twice daily to get relief from cough and cold	
Snake-bite	Powder of the seeds of *Moringa oleifera L.* mixed in tea to prepare a drink.	Fed the cows immediately at 15 minutes interval.
Dog Bite	Place the warm tea bag on wound to get relief from pain and swelling.	
Mouth sore	Drunk the animal a lot of healthy tea-drink thrice daily.	
Drowsiness	Drunk the animal a lot of healthy tea-drink at night.	
Adenomal intestine	Fed the fresh extract of green tea leaves to animals.	
Loss of hair/ Alopecia	Smear the green tea leaves extract once daily for 7 days.	
Senescence	Since green tea lowered the free radicals, so it act as antiageing under regular drinking.	
Liver Trouble/ colic pain	Mixing leaves extract of green tea, white tea in the drinking water of animals has been achieved desirable result.	
Conjunctivitis	Oil procured from leaves helps to cure tear fall.	
Weak-heart	Often tea consumption offers protection for healthy heart.	
Diabetes in dog	Regular intake of leaf leachate water controls diabetes and obesity.	
Foot rot of sheep	Immersed the feet for 15 minutes twice daily in the extract of leaves.	

Conclusion

The medicinal value of green tea are more than black tea. Besides it is a powerful antioxidant (Deng *et. al.*, 1998, Khan *et. al.*, 1992), anticancer agent (Dreosu *et al.*, 1997), sunstroke preventor, aids digestion (Khan *et. al.*, 1992) *etc.* As tea contains Mn, K so it prevents dental caries (Cao 1997). Tailoring of axillary flowers of tea defer senescence of leaves. Besides if the leaves are smeared by water hyacinth extract their senescence also delayed having evergreeness due to presence of gibberelic acid in water hyacinth.

3.8 Production of Biofertilizer Through Abatement of Sewage Pollution of Kolkata

Abstract

A study was carried out for proper utilization of various canals through collection of nutrients from waste water (sewage treatment) by *Eichhornia crassipes* and *Azolla pinnata*. Ca in general accumulates more in rhizome, Mg in roots and N_2 in leaves. The average results of the study carried out at different canals having industrial and domestic waste.

Keywords : *Sewage pollution, Eutrophication, Threshold level, biomass.*

Introduction

Kolkata, the most polluted city of Bengal. Though some corrective action was visible, forcing all vehicles to undergo pollution tests and ensure permissible pollutant levels. Similarly, will the sewage problem also dictate immediate action? Sewage has itself adversely affected the environment health. Every year come July, when the rains lash down in full monsoon fury, the city effluents leaks in every direction. Manholes and sewers get blocked, canals get flooded, roads waterlogged and the major canals which carry city generated sewage into the river Ganges are unable to cope with their overload. Keeping in view this new policy provides for recovery. Due to population pressure alongwith rise in unhygienic living standards may pose serious non biodegradable ecological problems in Kolkata causing detrimental effect to biotic system.

The accumulation capacity of water hyacinth and azolla for nutrients in the treatment of waste waters have gained considerable attention (Trivedy 1983). Though the chemical composition and accumulation of nutrients in these aquatic plants depends on the chemical nature of the habitat, season, position in stand etc.

The continued rise in cost of petroleum, the energy crisis, serious depletion of organic matter in tropical soils, ecologic and economic limitations of heavy use of chemical fertilizers have prompted in search for bio-fertilizers. As a biofertilizer both water hyacinth and *Azolla* are the traditional part of rice culture. Besides azolla is a water loving fern live in symbiosis with blue green algae (*Anabaena azollae*) are capable of fixing atmospheric nitrogen. To promoting these plants (within the fences nets of ½ Km to 10 Km) in a very large scale the numerous canals of Kolkata are the best site for farmers "to make the soil to serve the soil". Both these plants can be cultured in slow flowing water bodies like streams and canals. Flowing stress can be overcome by the application of phosphorous and GA_3 as foliar spray.

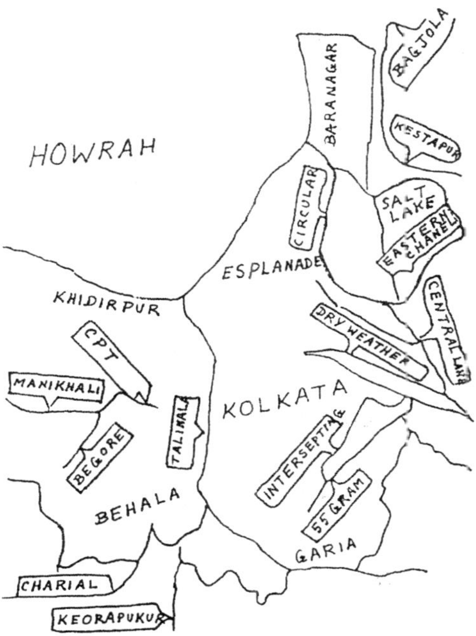

□ = Canals of Kolkata

Materials and Methods

The effect of sewage pollution on the growth performance was studied which were cultured in the canals and was compared with those cultured in the fresh water as control. The chlorophyll content from the leaves (10 mg) was measured spectrophotometrically according to Arnon (1949). After measuring the chlorophyll, the biomass by leaves was measured. The data were analysed from at least three/replicates and the whole experiment was calculated in two different years. Bitransplanting method of rice seedlings at 25 days intervals was followed to increase the yield.

Observations

Physico-chemical characteristic of waste water in different canals.

The physico-chemical characteristics of waste water in various canals used for growing water hyacinth and azolla are shown in Table. The pH of all the canals lie generally in between 7.5–7.8.

Table 6 : Biomass (mg/cm^2) and chlorophyll levels (in terms of OD values) of waterhyacinth and azolla

Plant Types	*Fresh Water (Control)*		*Polluted Water*	
	Biomass	*Chl*	*Biomass*	*Chl*
Water hyacinth	0.938	0.162	1.032	0.167
Azolla	1.126	0.113	1.157	0.128

The table shows that the plants occurring in the unpolluted sites with a low proportionate of chlorophyll and biomass.

Results and Discussion

Generally, polluted water may be capable of altering the aquatic ecosystem and reducing its biological productivity. The decline in dissolved oxygen concentration (Chawla *et. al.*, 1987) due to presence of heavy metals and detergents could impose detrimental effects. As both the plants are suitable for absorbing the polluted water to a threshold level and thereby purifying the water. So their biomass, chlorophyll and protein contents are higher compared to control plants. A stimulatory effect was observed instead of causing eutrophication. Safe levels for ecosystems and protocols for ecological safety evaluation of effluents and industrial chemical are lacking. This study suggests the importance of ecotoxicology in water quality maintenance and thereby meet the demand of green manure.

Aquatic plants, especially water hyacinth and azolla have been widely tried for the treatment of the waste water because of their tremendous capability of accumulating nutrients and other pollutants. However, still little attention is paid on them for their selective accumulation of nutrients. This characteristic is very effective to reduce the pollution in water and at the same time these plants are used as green manure, cattle and bird feed, soil condition etc. Due to heavy industrial and domestic wastes, considerable change in colour, odour, pH and chemical characteristic of the canals was observed.

3.9 Ancient Indigenous Abolishing Paddy Varieties of Bengal – An Observation

Although Charaka described 39 varieties of rice under 4 categories namely.

(*a*) *Sali* : Ripening in winter.

(*b*) *Shastika* : Ripening within 60 days in summer.

(*c*) *Vrihi* : Ripening in autumn and

(*d*) *Trinadhanya* : A wild varieties of food grains having awns.

Yet no attempt has been made to conserve the ancient indigenous abolishing paddy varieties of Bengal. Different varieties of rice differed from region to region. A country which has good potential available natural resources can overcome the problem of poverty alongwith gained prosperity. Crop improvement can be done by inoculating the desirable characters of native rice plants into the high yielding plants because the disease resistant natives plants can survive in drought area, saline soil, and in immersed as well as in flooded conditions etc. But the high yielding rice varieties have no such qualities. The straw of native plants are hardy, lusty and better for making thatched houses and food for domestic animals. Once upon a time more or less 6,000 varieties of paddy plants grown here and there in Bengal. Of them a few thousand varieties are donated to International Rice Research Institute of Philipines. Still no book is available covering the individual detail of desirable characteristic of 6000 varieties. From sincere observation during ethnobotanical survey it is found that undermentioned varieties are still grown here and there in restricted remote places.

List of Paddy Varieties

1. Ganga Pali.
2. Tulsi Mukul.
3. Tulsi Manjari.
4. Dahar Nagra.
5. Agnisal.
6. Sita Sal.
7. Asan Jharia.
8. Sundarmukhi.
9. Raghu Sal.
10. Vashamanik.
11. Churnakathi.
12. Darhkasal.
13. Balaram Sal.
14. Chandrakanta.
15. Mala.
16. Bahidkalamkathi.
17. Asan Latay.
18. Chakramala.
19. Dudenana.
20. Gobinda Bhog.
21. Bankchu.
22. Jhingesal.
23. Ram Sal.
24. Punjab Sal.
25. Dumurkandi.
26. Bau Bhog.
27. Vimsal.
28. Gour-Nitai.
29. Nagra Sal.
30. Laxmi Chura.

31. Haludgadhi.
32. Jalai.
33. Chali.
34. Lathisal.
35. Deradun.
36. Jwata.
37. Saru Patnai.
38. Jugal Dhan having 'twin endosperm' available only in the village Roport of Sonamukhi Block of Bankura District.
39. Kanakchur-Its parched-paddy has great demand to prepare sweetmeat of Joynagar in Sough 24 pgs. District.
40. Kashiphul
41. Drapodisal of Midnapore District.
42. Paramannesali or Hatipanjar of Murshidabad District.
43. Benaphul or Chiniskhakkar.
44. Boya-Suitable for water-lodged condition.
45. Mugibadam.
46. Kabirajsal its name itself reflects the folk belief that the rice serves as a Kabiraj and is fed to convalescing patients to quicken recovery.
47. Badshabhog.
48. Khudikhas or Bansphul (Scented rice of Birbhum District.
49. Kalidubarajpur.
50. Suryaujal
51. Tulaipanji (boiled rice are scented) of Dinajpur District.
52. Latasal.
53. Basudhan (*O. rufipogon* Griff)–Tribals use the grains as a supplement of rice.
54. Kuraghas (*Chloris variegata* SW.)–The perennial grass is used by the tribal as fodder and the watery juice of the

internodes as eyedrop against conjunctivitis, **though** it is not a paddy.

In undivided Bengal a list of native paddy varieties have available in the "Statistical Accounts of Bengal" by Willum Wilson Hunter. But within 150 years all the native rice plants are gradually being extinct.

Indigenous plants have good power of physiological adaptation, suitable for ecosystem, mixed cultivation, alongwith fish, duck and molluscs, tasty. Many of them (Tulaipanji, Gobindabhog etc.) are profitable than high yielding plant and grown well without manures and pesticides. They are not long-termed deleterious biological magnifier in ecological food chain. Genetically engineered plants are not safeful for food and environment.

3.10 Quick Regeneration of Stem Cuttings of Bamboos as Influenced by Planting Posture and IAA

Abstract

Investigation was made to determine the effect of IAA alongwith the planting posture on the regeneration of stem cutting of *Bambusa*. Very low concentrations of IAA (20 ppm) in horizontal posture show initiation of rooting after 10 days of application where as vertical posture with the same concentration of IAA takes 20 days for root initiation.

Keywords : *Culm, IAA, Horizontal posture, Inclined posture, Vertical posture, Sapling.*

Introduction

Raising of bamboo plants by cuttings in slanting posture (keeping an angle) is a common practice among the farmers but application of bioregulators and variation of posture may enhance the capacity of regeneration of stem cuttings. The process of regeneration is further to be affected by environmental factors *viz.* soil, light, temperature, humidity etc. Accurate planting posture is also essential for quick regeneration.

In the traditional way it is difficult to produce bamboo sapling. Though it is a monocarpic plant yet it is not grown from seeds. The objective of the present study was to promote reproductive capacity of bamboo plants. Since bamboo seeds are of rare occurrence and have their short period of viability.

Materials and Methods

Experiments were carried out during rainy season on cuttings of *Bambusa tulda* Roxb. of family poaceae in sand pit adjacent to Sonamukhi College. Plants were selected from Sonamukhi Forest Dept. From each plant 10 shoot pieces were selected for cuttings having 2–3 nodes containing culm buds. The aqueous solution of IAA were made and cuttings were dipped in hormonal solutions. Cuttings dipped in water were considered as control. Cuttings were planted at 3 postures (*viz.* vertical, inclined and horizontal). Four replicates each consisting of 3 stem cuttings were studied for each manipulation. Regular observations were made on regeneration of stem cuttings at 3 days interval. Spraying of water was done as and when required. The sprouted cuttings were transferred to the desired field. Through this process at a time numerous sapling can be evolved and may be distributed among the silvi-farmers.

Results and Discussion

All hormone treated stem cuttings show positive response of regeneration compared to control. Besides all horizontally placed cuttings of hormone treated and water treated (control) also sprouts faster than inclined and vertical. A significant rooting was observed in hormone treated cuttings when kept in horizontal posture. The regeneration pattern are as follows : horizontal > inclined > vertical.

Auxin has been found to stimulate rooting in stem cuttings of several plants. The quicker regeneration of culms in horizontal posture is due to the availability of balanced light, air and moisture from the sand.

Table 7 : Effect of IAA and Planting Posture on Sprouting of Culms

	Number of Days Required for Root Initiation				
Treatments	*5*	*10*	*15*	*20*	*25*
Control					
Vertical					+
Inclined				+	
Horizontal			+		
IAA					
Vertical				+	
Inclined			+		
Horizontal		+			

+ indicates root initiation time.

3.11 Allocation of Nerves on the Face

Investigation : Two pins or one pin

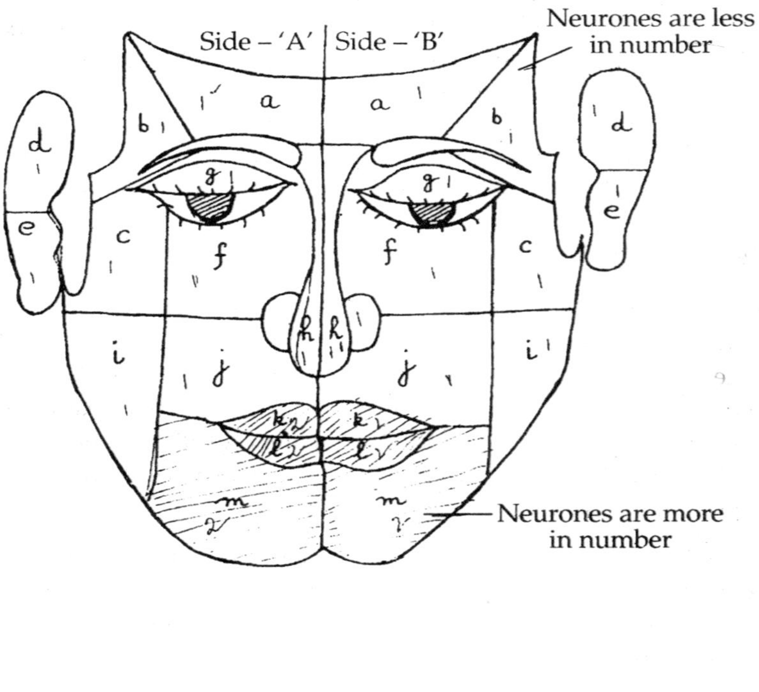

Instruction

Shade the zones where two pins are distinctly felt.

Questions

1. Does the distribution of sensory spots differ from person to person?
2. Does one half of the face differ from the other half?
3. Why do any two zones differ in their responses?
4. Propose a hypothesis to justify your explanation.
5. Propose an experiment to verify your hypothesis.

3.12 Allelopathic Susceptibility of Some Climbers in Their Community

Abstract

The work focuses on allelopathic susceptibility of some plants in their natural habitat. It enables the farmers to select appropriate site alongwith their effective supportable object.

***Keywords** : Allelopathic effect, Susceptibility, Cucurbitaceous, Inhibition.*

Introduction

Allelopathy is the detrimental effect of higher plants of 1 species (the donor) on the germination, growth or development of plants of another species, the recipient.[2] Fish-tail palm (*Caryota urens L*), *Carica papaya L.* (pepe), *Parthenium hysterophorus L*, *Thevetia nerifolia* Juss (kolkey) are the dominant species. Within their circumference sometimes farmers trying to cultivate climbers, but failed to achieve better yield. Besides these species are unpalatable to cattle due to presence of allelopathic chemicals. Since ancient time tribals observe these inhibitory plants.

Materials and Methods

For testing the allelopathic effect plants were grown in

close association with intact bamboos (which possess no allelopathic effect), fish-tail palms, *Parthenium*, papaya, kolkey. Besides extracts were prepared by crushing the shoot and root in a mixture with 100 ml of distilled water separately. Ten sterilized seeds of each plants were placed in petridishes (11 cm diameter) and were kept in room temperature, while seeds with distilled water were maintained as control separately. Seed germination and linear growth of plumule and radicle were also measured after 10 days.

Results and Discussions

The allelopathic effect of different concentrations of aqueous extracts from shoots and root of different plants were inhibitory to all parameters *viz.* seed germination, growth. Inhibition values calculated for seeds indicated that the inhibition increased progressively as the concentrations of extracts enhanced which is in conformity. Root extract of *Parthenium* was more inhibitory as compared to shoot extract of other plants. On the other hand 90% seed germination was recorded in the controlled condition. From the present findings it is evident that except bamboos all the experimental plants possess allelopathic chemicals which can not be used as supporters for raising cucurbitaceous climbers (*viz. Cucurbita*

Table 8 : Effect of Plant Extract (15%) on Seed Germination

Extract of plant species	*% of germination*	*Linear growth of Plumule (cm)*					
		Cururbita	*Lageneria*	*M. dioica*	*M. cochinchinensis*	*Dioscorea*	*Ipomoea*
Control	90	8.89±1.52	8.88±1.51	9.11±1.53	8.87+1.50	8.85±1.48	8.50±1.50
Bambusa	88	8.86±1.49	8.85±1.48	9.00±1.50	8.84±1.47	8.83±1.46	8.20±1.40
Caryota	45	5.85±1.40	5.84±1.39	5.82±1.38	5.86±1.41	5.88±1.42	5.89±1.41
Carica	55	6.00±0.97	4.35±0.83	6.20±0.98	6.30±0.99	6.11±0.97	6.10+0.98
Parthenium	40	5.80±1.35	5.81±1.36	5.20±1.10	5.10±1.20	5.86±1.40	5.81±1.30
Thevetia	42	6.90±1.04	6.17±0.99	6.99±1.05	7.20±1.70	7.10±1.60	7.30±1.80

All differences are significant at 1% level.

maxima Duch, Lageneria siceraria Mollina, Momordica dioica Roxb., M. cochinchinensis Spreng. (kakrol), Dioscorea pentaphyla L., (Dioscoreaceae), Ipomoea digitata L. (bhui kumra, Convolvulaceae).

These plants generally likes supports for their tendrils to hold the whole plants like firm grip against falling. Their tendrils are very sensitive in contact. They help the plant to climb up any other plant or object.

3.13 Skin Care Through Household Herbal Recipes or Remedies

Traditional preparations for natural beauty care contain several herbal recipes which have no side effect. Skin plays a vital role in our life. Everyone want to keep himself beautiful. Though the natural beauty of skin is achieved through balanced diet, mild exercise, stress free hygienic life, personalised home care and a healthy mental attitude. To ensuring youthful complexion eat lots of fresh fruits and green vegetables rich in vitamin A, C, E, which maintain the softness and smoothness of the skin texture. This study provides the following formulae on herbal recipes for the care of skin beauty.

***Keywords** : Herbal recipes, Ass milk, Cosmetic industry.*

Mix Turmeric (*Curcuma longa,* Zingiberaceae) paste and cream on the top of milk and then massage that mixture on the body.

Massage by equal quantities of cucumber (*Cucumis sativus,* Cucurbitaceae) and tomato (*Lycopersicum esculemtum,* Cucurbitaceae) juice. Shower after 10 minutes.

Massage the mixture of curd with wheat flour (*Triticum aestivum,* Gramineae) on the skin and then washed after 5 minutes.

Grind rose (*Rosa centifolia,* Rosaceae) petals and mixed with milk cream and apply to the skin followed by showering.

Spinach (*Spinacia oleracea,* Chenopodiaceae) and tomato juice mixture is supposed to be a good skin booster. Blend a tomato and bunch of spinach leaves in a mixie, dilute the mixture, add a pinch of salt and lime (*Citrus aurantifolia,* Rutaceae) to taste and used this healthy drink in every morning.

To get rid of pimples by applying garlic (*Allium sativum,* Liliaceae) extract alongwith honey or rub a cut onion (*Allium cepa,* Liliaceae) on your face. Besides pudina (*Mentha piperita,* Labiatae) leaves extract is good for preventing pimples.

For removing pimples or pox-scars make a paste of rice powder (*Oryza sativa*), lime juice alongwith curd or coconut milk and apply on the face regularly.

To get rid of from wart apply nailvarnish to it once daily until it dries up and falls off.

To get rid of from itching, rashes and allergies neem leachate water should be recommended as a daily dose for bath.

To avoid blackheads (mole) massage a paste of Khaus root or oil of vetiver (*Vetiveria zizanioides,* Gramineae), lime juice and coconut milk daily till disappear.

To achieve soft beautyness cut beet root (*Beta vulgaris,* Chenopodiaceae) into small pieces and grind then. Extract or squeeze juice from beet root and massage to your face for 5 minutes daily. Shower after 10 minutes with mild soap or gram flour (*Cicer arietinum,* Papilionaceae).

Mixed sandal wood (Swet chandan-*Santalum album,* Santalaceae) with rose water and add 4–5 drops of ass milk in it and apply on the face and body. Shower after 15 minutes with warm water.

Lemon (*Citrus reticulata,* Rutaceae) juice mixed with warm honey massage on the face and wash after it dries.

Massage the skin with ass milk like the queen Juleo Chemny of Denmark who applied this for 38 years to sustain her beauty till death as she discovered it is a good natural moisturiser.

Grate carrot (*Daucus carota,* Umbelliferae) and boil. Massage that mixture in the body to get fairy skin.

Discussion

Formulation for cure of complexion brightener can be prepared from herbs. The herbs mentioned above cover a number of skin-general body complaints, providing natural colour and nutrients to the body. Ayurvedic texts contain several recipes, which may be applied in cosmetic industry. So, there is a lot of scope for research on herbs for natural colour of the skin.

3.14 Remarkable Abolishing Sand-Binding Plants of Coastal Area in Bengal

Abstract

The study reflects on the naturally available abolishing sand-binders which may reduces the wave, wind-blow, soil erosion and denudation of plant cover as well as attract the tourist and naturalist.

Keywords : Sand-binder, Soil erosion, Bio-diversity, Sand dune.

Introduction

Removal of top fertile soil by certain abiotic agents like water, wind etc. has a detrimental affect on coastal life. So species formation is necessary. Under the sand dune stabilization scheme, mulching of dunes (spreading straw, rotting leaves or plastic sheeting over sand dune-as a protective layer) has given priority. This has also been followed by planting and subsequent management of naturally available suitable sand-binding species of plants like *Acacia tortilis* (Israeli Babul) and grasses. Here polyculture is more effective than monoculture. Plants of this beach have a tendency to grow small with restricted growth.

Soil erosion is a natural process and it is neither new nor necessarily alarming except when it outpaces the formation of new soil. It takes approximately 500 to 1000 years for an inch of the top layer to build up. But soil erosion is one of the most difficult problems faced by the coastal regions of Digha, Mandermoni, Junput etc., where the eroded soil, threatens the life span of living beings. Generally sand-building plants stabilize loose soil and detritus and act as a filter for land runoffs and function as a bullwork against sea erosion and protect the hinterland from cyclonic storms and high velocity winds. Rao (1986) mentioned their major roles :

(*a*) Help in soil formation by trapping debris.

(*b*) Provide appropriate eco-system. Keeping in view to overcome the soil erosion the present survey has been made.

Materials and Methods

During ecological survey (2002–2004) about biodiversity on behalf of our eco-club we observed some sand binding plants. Plant specimens were collected from the study area, authenticated and kept in the herbarium for future. Plants were collected from Vitarkanika, Chandbali, Chandaneswar and Talsari of Orissa State and also from Udoypur, Digha, Junput and Mandarmani of W. Bengal, Vitarkanika → Chandbali → Puri → Konarok → Talsari → Udoypur → Digha → Shankarpur → Mandarmani. The total length of the route from Vitarkanika to Mandarmani is 740 km.

Results and Discussion

The removal of top soil by violent wind is a common phenomenon to those areas which are dry and devoid of any form of vegetation except in few places. It is has been noted that 0.1 million hectares (approx.) of beach have been subjected to wind erosion.

The best method to conserve the soil is bringing the sand-dune under vegetation cover. This can be done through growing grasses, shrubs and trees of such types :

1. ***Myriostachya wightiana* Nees, Pani Ghas, Fam :** Poaceae, Gregarious perennial grass. Its long wiry flexible roots are used for cordage.
2. ***Saccharum spontaneum* L. Kash, Fam :** Poaceae.
3. ***Spinifex squarrosus* L. Seashore Grass, Fam :** Poaceae. Scarcely found on the sand-dunes of Bay of Bengal.

4. ***Carex indica*** **L. Slough Grass, Fam :** Cyperaceae. Found on sandy places and are very efficient in binding sand.
5. ***Ipomoea biloba*** **Forsk. Goats' Foot, Fam :** Convolvulaceae. The leaves of which resemble the hoofs of a goat, is a sand-binder found on sea-shore.
6. ***Ipomoea pes-caprae*** **Sweet, Fam :** Convolvulaceae.
7. ***Casuarina equisetifolia*** **Forst, Beef-wood tree (Banjhau), Fam :** Casuarinaceae. A common tall tree.
8. ***Prosopis juliflora*** **(Bilati babla), Fam :** Mimosaceae. Having deep root system that can tap deep moisture supplies or go dormant during dry conditions. It becomes a condensed bush in an undisturbed site. But it takes the shape of a tree when its lower branches are cut down.
9. ***Vetiveria zizanioides*** **(Linn.), Khas-Khas, Bena, Fam :** Poaceae. A densely tufted grass upto 180 cm high, rhizome aromatic, culms stout and rigid. Dried roots are made into mats and hung over window during summer.
10. ***Eragrostis cynosuroides*** **Beauv., Kush, Fam :** Poaceae, used in religious ceremonies. In submerged condition they can survive.
11. ***Bambusa bambos*** **L. Willd (Spiny), Bans, Poaceae :** It can increases the water-holding capacity, check soil erosion and makes the soil fertile by its abscised leaves.

Soil erosion by winds is very common in these areas where there is not enough vegetation to cover and protect the soil. Such a condition obtain along the sand shores of Bay of Bengal. Here sand is constantly blown up from one place to another during summer. Anything like agricultural fields which lie in the path of the wind are covered with sand and become unproductive in course of time. Plants get buried in the sand and are destroyed for ever. Only the above species of grasses, shrubs and trees are capable of growing in such coastal areas. They are, therefore, called "sand binders" and are acting as stabilizers of wind and sea wave action along the coastal belts as well as a buffer against the oil-slicks washed down from the seas.

Though naturally grown *Ipomoea biloba* and *Spinifex* sps found abundant in Orissa beach and Mandarmani beach but they are absent in the beaches of Digha, Junput etc., specially the *Spinifex* sps due to human interference.

Indiscriminate and unregulated use of vegetative cover leads to ecological imbalance. The balance can be brought back only by creating harmonious relationship between man and nature. This is possible only by scientific cultivation of the various types of sand binding plants.

3.15 Study of Ecoflame in Black Variety of *Capsicum annuum* L. (Family Solanaceae)

Abstract

Black chillis have great economic importance in West Rarrh due to their better yield, pungent smell and taste. These plants under the specialized edaphic factors exhibits ecoflame which have ecological importance as the cultivators are quite ignorant about this even why their black varieties converted to whitish or palish.

Introduction

Turesson (1932) regarded the ecotype as an adaptation to the local habitat. Even if individuals of one ecotype are transplanted in a changed habitat, the original characteristics persist as long as the plant survive in a changed environment. So, Ecotypes are the races or the product of the reaction between the genotype and the habitat. Ecotypes are genetically fixed. In this field, Turesson's experiment may be regarded as pioneer. He is familiar with the phenomenon of the different environmental tolerances of various species, and that different populations of the same species occupying distinctive habitats frequently showed morphological and physiological traits, often of an adaptive nature.

Turesson's observed the reactions of the plants in cultivations over the years in terms of habit, height, flowering time, etc. and found that in some cases the differences noted between populations in the field disappeared, in other cases showed intergradations, but in most instances persisted. These persistent differences therefore appeared to be due to genetic differences and that the genetically different races were often correlated with the habitat differences. Besides some plants under the specialized condition differ in appearance, but these variations are not genetically fixed and when transplanted by Turessions to his garden under neutral condition, the variation vanished. This apparent variation are called in ecological term, ecoflame. To observe this ecoflame philic phenomena the black chillis are found to be suitable and at the same time the objective of this study is to screen the genetically fit plants due to action of the species and the habitat.

Materials and Methods

Certified seeds of *Capsicum annuum* were surface sterilized in 0.1% $HgCl_2$ for 1 minute and then washed well in running water. These were shown in the first week of November in an experimental seed-bed ($1m^2$) containing loamy soil mixed with rotted farmyard manure for raising seedings. At the age of 21 days seedlings were transplanted in 3 experimental plots (loamy, lateritic, sandy soil) in parallel lines with a gap of 45 cm between rows and 30 cm. between plants. All the experimental plots

Table 9

No. of Sps.	*Treatments*			
	Loamy Soil	*Lateritic Soil*	*Sandy Soil*	*Remarks*
White or Normal variety of chilli	Leaf, flower, pod is white	Leaf, flower, pod is white	Leaf, flower pod is white	Ecotype (*i.e.* genetically fixed)
Black variety of chilli	Leaf, flower, pod is blackish	Leaf, flower, pod is blackish	Leaf, flower pod is whitish	Ecoflame (*i.e.* modification of genes)

Table showing the comparative study of 2 species.

were done in a net house to avoid damage from pests. The soil between the lines was transferred around the plants in such a way that the plants were ultimately raised on straight ridges. Appropriate watering was done between this ridges as and when required. *i.e.* care was taken to keep the soil drenched up to the time of harvest. Transplant experiments are performed in order to decide whether variations are heritable or non-heritable and reversible, a dual approach is employed.

Results and Discussion

From the above mentioned result it is found that normal variety of chillis are genetically fixed while the black varieties of chilli when transplanted on sandy soil they exhibits ecoflame as their phenotypical black character is being vanished within a month. If it is replanted in loamy soil (*i.e.* neutral one) from the sandy one the black colours reappear *i.e.* the differences will disappear which support the view of Turesson 1925; Clausen *et. al.*, 1948. Sandy soils are the initiator of ecoflame as they are light, loose, poor in both nutrients and water retaining capacity; and as such, they dry up quickly and become heated in sun light compared to loamy and lateritic soil. Cultivation of plants of uniform heredity in varied environmental conditions so as to show the effect of different environments on the same genotype. Lastly it is concluded with the Odum's (1971) remarks that "organisms are not just 'slaves' of the physical environment; they adapt themselves and modify the physical environment so as to reduce the limiting effects of physical conditions of existence."

References

1. Chattopadhay, A. and M. Maji 1976. Poor Man's Medicine, Man and life 2 : 126.
2. Ghosh A 2004. Natural biocides and biofertilizers. Natural Product Radiance. 3 : 173.
3. Cox PA (1994). In Chadwick D.J. Marsh J. (Eds) Ethnobotany and the Search of New Drugs, John Wiley and Sons. England 25-36.
4. Ghosh A. (2002). Ethnoveterinary medicines from the tribal areas of Bankura and Medinipur districts, West Bengal, IJTK 1 : 93-95.

5. Ghosh A. (2003). Herbal folk remedies of Bankura and Medinipur districts, West Bengal. IJTK 2 : 393-396.

6. Jain SK. (1963), Observations on ethnobotany of tribals of Madhya Pradesh. Vanyajati 11 : 177-183.

7. Jain SK. De Jn (1964). Some less known plant foods among the tribal of Purulia (West Bengal). Science and Culture. 30 : 825-286.

8. Jain SK (1989). Ethnobotany : an interdisciplinary science for holistic approach to man plant relationships. In : Jain SK (ed.) Methods and approaches in ethnobotany. Society of ethnobotany, Lucknow, Uttar Pradesh : 9-12.

9. Kar B (1999). Report on ethnomedicinal uses of *Gloriosa superba* in Bankura district of West Bengal, India. Geobios New Reports. 8(2) : 135-136.

10. Ghosh A, Plant and clay dyes used by weavers and potters in West Bengal, Nat. Pro. Rad, 2004, 3(2), 91.

11. Roy A, Moktan B and Sarkar PK, Traditional technology in preparing legume-based fermented foods of Orissa, IJTK, 2007, 6(1), 12–16.

12. Gokhale SB, Tatiya AV, Bakliwal SR and Fursule RA, Natural dye yielding plants in India, Nat. Pro. Rad. 2004 3(4), 228–233.

13. Gaur RD, Traditional dye yielding plants of Uttarakhand, India, Nat pro. Rad, 2008, 7(2), 154–165.

14. Ghosh AK, Ethnobiology : Therapeutics and Natural Resources, Daya Publishing House, Delhi, 2009.

15. Arnon DI, Copper enzymes in isolated chloroplasts. Polyphenol oxidase in *Beta vulgaris*. Plant Physiol, 1949, 24, 1–15.

16. Nishida K and Kabayashi K, Dyeing properties of natural dyes from vegetable sources, Am Dyestuff Rep, 1992, 81(9), 26.

17. Mathpal Y, rock Art in Kumaon Himalaya, Indira Gandhi National Centre for the Arts and Arryan Book International, New Delhi, 1995.

18. Siddiqui, S.A. 2004. Lac–The Versatile natural resin. Natural Product Radiance. 3(5) : 332–337.

19. Cao J, Observation of caries incidence among a tea drinking population. J Dental Health, 1997, 31, 86–89.

20. Deng ZY, Tao BY, Xiaolin L, Jinming H and Yifeng C, Effect of green tea and black tea on blood glucose triglycerides and antioxidants in aged rat. J. Agric Food Chem, 1998, 46, 3875–3878.

21. Devi DB, Singla A and Boparai R, Tea-Role in health in and diseases. J. Nat Pro Rad, 2004, 3(3), 156–166.

22. Dreosu IE, Wargovich MJ and Yang CS, Inhibition of carcinogenesis by Tea : the evidence from experimental studies. Crit Rev Food Sci Nutr, 1997, 37, 761–770.

23. Karawya MS, Abdel Wahab SM, El Olemy MM and Farrag NM, Diphenylamine and antihyperglycemic agent from onion and tea, J. Nat Prod, 1984, 47, 775–780.

24. Khan SG, Katiyar SK, Aggarwal R and Mukhtar H, Enhancement of antioxidant and phase II enzymes by oral feeding of green tea polyphenols in drinking water to SKH-1 hairless mice; possible role in canels chemoprevention, cancer Res, 1992, 52(14), 4050–4052.

25. Kreydijyeh SI, Abdel-Hasan Baydoum E and Churukian ZM, Tea extract inhibits intestinal absorption of glucose and sodium in rats. Comp Biochem physiol C pharmacol Toxical Endocrinol 1994, 108, 359–365.

26. Sharma G, Tea as a health drink, In : The Tribune-Chandigarh, India, Nov. 6, 2000.

27. Stensvold I, Tverdal A, Solvoll K and Foss OP, Tea Consumption : relationship to cholesterol blood pressure, and coronary and total mortality, prev Med, 1992, 21, 546–553.

28. Thelle DS, Coffee, tea and coronary heart disease, Curr Opin Lipidol, 1995, 6, 25–27.

29. Arnon, D.I. : Copper enzymes in isolated chloroplast, Polyphenol oxidase in *Beta vulgaris*. Plant Physiol. 24 : 1–15 (1949).

30. Trivedy, R.K. : Water hyacinth for control, biogas, paper pulp, animal feed and manure. Environ and Ecol. 1 : 139–141 (1983).

31. Chawla G., Viswanathan, P.N. and Devi, S. : Biochemical studies on the toxicity of linear alkylbenzene sulphonate to *Scenedesmus quardicauda* in culture. Environ. Exp. Bot. 27 : 311–323 (1987).

32. Hunter WW, 1864, Statistical Accounts of Bengal.

33. Ramiah K and Ghosh RL, 1980, Origin and distribution of cultivated plants of S.E. Asia, Journal of Genetics and Plants Breeding, Vol. XI-XIII (1951-1953). pp. 7–13; ICAR, New Delhi, pp. 271–272.

34. Nanda KK and Kochhar VK, Vegetative propagation of plans. Kalyani Pub., New Delhi, 1985, 123–193.

35. Pal D., Gupta S.K., Afroz N and Singh C., Regeneration of stem cuttings of *Nerium oleander* L. as influenced by IAA and planting posture. Adv. Plant Sci., 1988, I (2), 219–222.

36. Prasad A, A note on the vegetative propagation of medicinal plants. Curr. Sci., 1962, 31, 202–203.

37. Torrey JG, Root hormone and plant growth. Ann Rev Plant Physiol, 1976, 27, 435–459.

38. Anonymous, The Wealth of India : Raw Materials, CSIR, New Delhi, Vol. 1–X, 1048–1976.

39. Narwal SS, Allelopathy in Crop Production, Scientific Publishers, Jodhpur, India, 1994.

40. Rice EL, Allelopathy (2nd ed.) Academic Press, Inc., Orianda, Florida, 1984.

41. Khanna A (2002). Plants in Beauty Care and Beauty Products. Recent progress in Medicinal Plants. Vol. – 3, Aesthetics (Editors V.K. Singh, J.N. Govil and Gurdip Singh), SCI Tech Publishing. USA, pp. 89–120.

42. Rao TA and Mukherjee A.K., Ecological aspects along shores of Burabalanga tidal estuary, Orissa State. *Ibid.,* 1971, 76(B), 201–206.

43. Rao TA and Sastry ARK, An ecological approach towards classification of coastal vegetation of India-I. Strand Vegetation. Ind. For 1972, 98, 597–607.

44. Roa TA and Sastry ARK, An ecological approach towards classification of coastal vegetation of India-II. Estuarine vegetation. *Ibid.,* 1974, 100, 438–452.

45. Rao TA and Sastry ARK, An outline of the coastal vegetation of India. Bull Bot Surv India, 1977, 16, 101–115.

46. Clausen, J., Keck, D.D. and Hiesey, W.M. 1948. Experimental studies on the nature of species, III. Environmental responses of climatic races of *Achillea.* Carnegic Inst. Wash. Publ. 581.

47. Turesson G. 1925. The plant species in relation to habitat and climate– Contributions to the knowledge of genecological units. Hereditas 6:147–236.

48. Turesson, G. 1932. Die Pflanzenart als Klimaindikator. Kungi, Physiogr. Sallsk. i. Lund. Forhandl. Z. No. 4.

49. Odum, E.P. 1971. Fundamentals of Ecology. W.S. Saunders Company, Philadelphia and London.

4

Regulation of Senescence

4.1 Regulation of Senescence of Rice (*Oryza* sativa CV. *Jaya*) by Hormones and Nutrients

Prior to harvest, the levels of chlorophyll in the leaves of manipulated plants of *Oryza sativa* L. cv Jaya was higher than control plants indicating the order of senescence as control > GA_3 > water hyacinth.

Keywords *: Senescence, Foliar spray, Dry weight.*

Available literature shows that only a few stray attempts have been made to study the effect of foliar nutrients[1] applied as foliar sprays to correlate the longevity of plants alongwith yields. The present investigation aims at analysing the effects of hormones and nutrients on growth and longevity of rice plant (cv. Jaya) when these are applied at different developmental stages of the plant.

Certified seeds of Jaya were surface sterilized in 0.1% $HgCl_2$ for 1 minute and then washed well in running water. These were sown in experimental plot for raising seedlings. At the age of 21 days, seedlings were transplanted with one seedling per earthenware pot containing loamy soil previously mixed with organic farmyard manure. Watering was done as and when required.

Aqueous solution (100 mg/l) of gibberellic acid (GA_3) and water hyacinth extracts were separately prepared using 0.5% teepol as surfactant. Each solution was sprayed at the rate of 3 ml per plant at the 3 developmental stages, *viz.* seedling (plant age 48 days), pre-flowering (plant age 80 days) and post-flowering (plant age 96 days). Spraying was executed consecutively for 4 days in the morning to avoid scorching. Each time control plants were sprayed with equal amount of 0.5% teepol. Chlorophyll levels were estimated from randomized leaf samples following to Arnon's[2] method. For determination of dry weight, plants were oven dried at 70°C for 72 hours.

All the manipulated plants contained higher levels of chlorophyll and dry weight (Table 1) than controls. The levels of chlorophyll in the leaves and dry weight of different plants are as follows : Waterhyacinth > GA_3 > Control. Whole plant senescence is therefore delayed by hormones and nutrients. Plants treated with waterhyacinth extracts and GA_3 deferred senescence of leaves and increased the economic yield due to a balanced nutrient exhaustion out of the source organ. Due to accumulation Ca, Mg and N in leaves of water-hyacinth (*Eichhornia crassipes* Solms), foliar spray of water-hyacinth extract on rice induces luxurient growth as water-hyacinth have effective capability of accumulating nutrients.

Table 1 : Chlorophyll Content (mg/g freshweight), Dry Weight (g Plant) of Randomized Leaf and Plant Samples at 3 Developmental Stages

Treatments	*Senescence Parameters*	*Seedling (48 days old)*	*Pre-flowering (80 days old)*	*Post-flowering (96 days old)*
Control	Chlorophyll	5.55	5.25	4.81
	Dry wt.	355.8	381.4	411.1
GA_3	Chlorophyll	5.64	4.38	4.96
	Dry wt.	369.1	391.2	419.3
Water-hyacinth	Chlorophyll	5.7	5.3	4.97
	Dry wt.	380	399	420
CD at 5%	Chlorophyll	0.06	0.18	0.09
	Dry wt.	7.50	9.05	5.67

4.2 Natural Antioxidants are the Precursor of Anti-ageing

O_2-free radicals induce tissue damage thereby it may

causes a number of ailments. Antioxidants minimize the effect of free radicals through different ways and may prevent the animals from various ailments. Antioxidants may be of natural or synthetic. Some synthetic antioxidants have deleterious effect on human body. So, search for potential antioxidants are necessary to delayed the senescence of human. There is a need to incorporate antioxidants in the diet. The possible use of naturally available antioxidant rich plants are documented in the present paper for human well being. Though gerontologists want to retard the senescence process through life-saving food and beverages. Generally nutritionally adequate somewhat deficient in calories full of antioxidants food and beverage intake delayed the senescence process.

Introduction

Some food and beverages have free radical scavenging properties (Ghosh 2005) due to presence of appropriate level of antioxidants. Antioxidants act cat by scavenging reactive O_2, by inhibiting their formation, by binding transition metal ions and preventing formation of OH and/or decomposition of lipid hydroperoxides, by repairing damage or by any combination of the above (Niwa *et. al.*, 2001). An antioxidant is any substance that when present at low concentrations significantly delays or prevents oxidation of cell content like carbohydrates, proteins, fats and DNA. Mn, Cu, Zn, Selenium, Vitamin E, C, albumin, carotenoids, flavonoids, β-carotene etc. are as scavenger. Generally 'oxidative stress' results from a series of events which deregulates the cellular functions and leads to various ailments, *viz.* ageing, arthritis, asthma, AIDS, cardiovascular problems, diabetes, cataract, liver disorder, alzheimer's disease, retinopathy etc. (Tiwari 2001).

Materials and Methods

Antioxidant activities of various food and beverages calculated by using the ferric reducing antioxidant power assay (FRAP assay). Besides, antioxidant potency were also determined by estimating superoxide dismutase activity (SOD) and catalase activity.

Results and Discussion

National dietary antioxidants like vitamin 'C', 'E', β-carotene etc. enhanced life if daily eating properly in hygienic way with balanced diet. Generally with the advent of ageing some deleterious products accumulates within the cells accelerate senescence. All the plants mentioned are having vitamin ('C', 'E', carotenoids etc.), flavonoids, polyphenols possess remarkable antioxidant activity which is neither restricted to a particular part of the plant. In nature there are wide variety of naturally occurring antioxidants which differ in composition, properties, mechanism and site of action. So, need further research for exploring their antioxidant potential alongwith how one can survive for a long time in the earth which is a latent dream of everybody.

A brief description of the common antioxidant plants is documented below :

Sl. No.	*Botanical Name*	*Vernacular Name*	*Family*	*Part used*
1.	*Allium sativum* L.	Rasun	Liliaceae	Bulb
2.	*Asparagus racemosus* Willd.	Satamuli	–do–	Shoot
3.	*Bryonia alba* L.	Bryony	Cucurbitaceae	Root
4.	*Cinnamomum zeylanicum* Breyn	Dalchini	Lauraceae	Bark
5.	*Curcuma longa* L.	Halud	Zingiberaceae	Rhizome
6.	*Daucus carota* L.	Gajor	Apiaceae	Root
7.	*Emblica officinalis* Gaertn.	Amlaki	Euphorbiaceae	Fruit
8.	*Foeniculum vulgare* Mill.	Mouri	Apiaceae	Fruit oil
9.	*Garcinia kowa* Roxb.	Kaglichu	Guttiferae	Fruit (aril)
10.	*Ginkgo biloba* L.	Ginkgo	Ginkgoaceae	Leaf
11.	*Glycyrrhiza glabra* L.	Jastimadhu	Fabaceae	Root
12.	*Lavandula angustifolia* Mill.	Lavender	Lamiaceae	Aerial part
13.	*Lycopersicon esculentum* Mill.	Bilati begun	Solanaceae	Fruit
14.	*Mangifera indica* L.	Am	Anacardiaceae	Tender leaf, Fruit

(Contd...)

Sl. No.	Botanical Name	Vernacular Name	Family	Part used
15.	*Momordica charantia* L.	Karala	Cucurbitaceae	Fruit, Leaf
16.	*Murraya koenigii* (L.) *Spreng*	Currypata	Rutaceae	Leaf
17.	*Ocimum sanctum* L.	Krishnatulsi	Lamiaceae	–do–
18.	*Piper nigrum* L.	Golmarich	Piperaceae	Fruit
19.	*Plantago asiatica* L.	Isabgul	Plantaginaceae	Seed
20.	*Prunus domestica* L.	Plum	Rosaceae	Fruit
21.	*Santalum album* L.	Chandan	Santalaceae	Heart wood
22.	*Solanum melongena* L.	Begun	Solanaceae	Fruit
23.	*S. tuberosum* L.	Alu	–do–	Tuber
24.	*Swertia chirayita* Ham.	Chirata	Gentianaceae	Whole plant
25.	*Withania somnifera* Dun.	Ashwagandhya	Solanaceae	Root
26.	*Zingiber officinale* Rosc.	Ada	Zingiberaceae	Rhizome

4.3 Source-Sink Relationship During Monocarpic Senescence of *Pachyrhizus angulatus* (Papilionaceae and *Papaver somniferum* (Papaveraceae)

Abstract

In control plants of *Pachyrhizus angulatus* having storage root and reproductive sink organs, the plants senesced earlier (as determined by the loss of chlorophyll) as compared to those of deflorated and deshooted ones. At harvest the dry weight of storage roots was achieved in the order : deshooted > deflorated > normal. Prior to harvest in *Papaver somniferum,* the levels of chlorophyll and protein in the leaves of defruited was higher than deflorated or control indicating the senescence pattern as control > deflorated > defruited. Evidently, the presence of latex alongwith seeds is more lethal than that of flowers.

Keywords : *Chlorophyll, storage root, reproductive sink organs, defruited, deflorated, dry weight.*

Introduction

Working with a number of crop plants some authors have opined that senescence of monocarpic plants is species specific or even varietal. Despite the present knowledge about the role of roots for the supply of cytokinin to the shoot as well as for the diversion of nutrient from other organs (in case of storage root), the crucial role of such organs, separately or in combination with reproductive sink, has not been worked out. *Pachyrhizus angulatus* seems to be ideal for studying the role of reproductive sink as well as storage roots, as both are present in a single or in different plant system and may contribute for the manipulation of senescence syndrome.

Source-sink related whole plant senescence has been widely studied on several agricultural crops which produce harvestable fruits/seeds of great economic importance, as the plants die abruptly after maturation, it is logical to conclude that both developing flowers and fruits play a vital role in the determination of senescence. As flowers cause a little withdrawal as compared to the capsules (containing latex) while contributing senescence inducing substance to the leaf (Noodén, 1980), the study of the roles of the two reproductive structures separately or in combination seem rewarding in elucidating process. *Papaver somniferum* may provide useful information for the determination of source-sink related mechanism of senescence.

Materials and Methods

Surface-sterilized and water-soaked seeds of *Pachyrhizus angulatus* were sown in the field in the first week of November in parallel lines with a gap of 45 cm between rows and 25 cm between plants. Sprinkling of water was done on the seed bed at regular intervals until seed germination. Formation of storage root initiated at the plant age of 35 days. Defloration was performed on 20 plants at the age of 50 days (flower-initiation stage) and continued until no more flowers appeared in order to modify the source and sink capacities. In order to get better yield tailoring of partial aerial shoots were conducted on 20 plants. Non-excised plants served as control. For the study of senescence and source-sink relationship chlorophyll, sugar, dry weight of whole plants were determined at the age of 85 days.

Certified seeds of *Papaver somniferum* were procured from Bhubaneswar, Government of Orissa. Seeds were surface sterilized in 0.1% $HgCl_2$ for 1 minute and then washed well in running water. Seeds were sown at the advent of winter in the field in lines on the ridges (30 × 30 cm apart). Soils were kept moist lateritic previously mixed with rotted farmyard manure. Watering was done as and when required.

Physical manipulation were conducted on 20 plants where flowers were pinched off at the age of 40 days and the process continued till flowers appeared (plant age 75 days). In another 20 plants, capsules were removed until their final setting. Non-excised plants served as control. For the assessment of senescence and source-sink relationship, chlorophyll, protein of leaves alongwith dry weight of plants were estimated at the age of 105 days. The chlorophyll was extracted from 50 mg randomized samples of leaves with chilled acetone (–4°C) and the values were determined at 660 nm in a spectrochem spectrophotometer according to Arnon (1949). After removing the chlorophylls the same samples were washed 3 times with trichloroacetic acid (18%) and the residue dissolved in 1 ml of 0.5 M NaOH at 85°C for 1 h. After removing the tissue debris, the protein was estimated with the Folin-phenol reagent (Lowry *et al.*, 1951). For the estimation of dry weight, the aerial parts and the respective plant parts were oven-dried at 80°C for 12 h. Extraction of soluble sugar was done from the oven-dried (at 80°C for 12 h) and powdered randomized samples of leaves as collected for chlorophyll estimation. The plant material alongwith 5 ml glass-distilled water was autoclaved (15 lbs pressure) for 15 minutes and then centrifuged at 10,000 g for 10 min. The supernatant was used for the estimation of soluble sugar with 0.2% anthrone reagent (McCready *et al.*, 1950). Data were statistically analysed by taking the source of variances as days, replication and error. The C.D. (critical difference) values were calculated (Panse and Sukhatme, 1967) at the significance level P = 0.05.

Results and Discussion

In *P. angulatus*, the different plants having variation of

storage root show differential behaviour in response to the development of senescence. Storage roots therefore play a vital role in the deferment of senescence. This is due to the supply of cytokinin from the storage root to the leaves in general and particularly to the nearest leaf (Ghosh and Biswas, 1991). The chlorophyll of the leaves of deflorated plants was higher than those of control plants but lower than the partially deshooted ones indicating the pattern of senescence as control > deflorated > partially deshooted (Table 2). The maximum deferment of

Table 2 : The levels of chlorophyll, sugar and dry weight of *P. angulatus* at the age of 85 days (just prior to harvest).

Treatments	*Chlorophyll* *mg/g FW*$^{-1}$	*Sugar* *mg/g DW*$^{-1}$	*Dry weight* *g/plant*$^{-1}$
Control	0.67	265	30.2
Deflorated	0.85	225	32
Deshooted	1.05	205	33.1
CD at 5%	0.15	12.1	0.65

leaf senescence in partially deshooted plants is due to the absence of flowers which might supply the senescence signal (Ghosh and Biswas, 1995) through downward migration for the induction of senescence of the leaves and at the same time supply of cytokinin by the storage root. Besides there is a direct correlation between sugar level and senescence. Highest increase of storage roots again indirectly support the predominant role for the supply of cytokinin and to increase the longevity of plants.

In *P. somniferum*, the control plants senesced earlier than the excised plants. The chlorophyll level of defruited plants remained higher than those of deflorated and control plants indicating the order of senescence as control > deflorated > defruited (Table 2). Maximum deferment of senescence in both deflorated and defruited plants is due to absence of flower, fruits and latex which might supply the senescence signal (Biswas and Mandal, 1987). Noodén (1980, 1984), Ghosh and Biswas (1995) and Ghosh (2002) also concluded that senescence signals development from the flowers and fruits migrated downwards for the induction of leaf senescence. After exudation of latex by incision from the capsules the senescence is delayed. So the latex also plays a prominent role in senescence. Maximum increase in dry weight was found in defruited plants which again indirectly supports the predominant role of fruits along with latex for the longevity of plants.

Table 3 : The level of chlorophyll, protein and dry weight of *P. somniferum* at the age of 105 days (just prior to harvest)

Treatments	*Chlorophyll mg/g FW^{-1}*	*Protein mg/g FW^{-1}*	*Dry weight g/plant^{-1}*
Control	0.84	39	19
Deflorated	1.00	41.2	20
Delatexed	1.02	41	21
Defruited	1.07	40.8	22
CD at 5%	0.15	4.15	0.66

4.4 Correlative Senescence in *Helianthus annuus* L. During Reproductive Maturation

Abstract

In normal control plant (*Helianthus annuus*) having large capitulum, all the leaves senesced (as determined by the loss of chlorophyll) earlier compared to small capitulum. In both the set, the 1st leaf from the top senesced earlier (non-sequential) compared to that of 3rd leaf, but the reverse (sequential) was found in plant lacking seeds (hot-water treatment). The level of chlorophyll decreased in the 3rd leaf of the plant, when the same subtended a lateral shoot. Seed weight also decreased when the plants subtended a lateral shoot. The results emphasized the more deleterious effect of "senescence signal" than the nutrient exhaustion in these plants.

Keywords : *Capitulum, Chlorophyll, Sequential.*

Introduction

Source-sink related whole plant senescence has been widely studied on several agricultural annual crops (Biswas and Chaudhuri 1980; Biswas and Ghosh 1989). As the plants die after reproductive maturation, it is logical to conclude that developing fruits play a vital role in the determination of foliar senescence. The role of flowers and fruits has been speculated by Choudhuri and Mondal (1988) and also observed by the present author that flowers are more lethal than the fruits for the development of whole plant senescence.

A great deal of information has been available on the post harvest physiology of cut-flowers of several horticultural plants (Whitehead and Halevy 1989), but very little is known about the role of reproductive propagules on the mechanism of senescence of such plant in intact condition. As flowers caused little withdrawal compared to the fruits, while contributing the senescence inducing substance to the leaf (Nooden 1984).

The study of the roles of the two reproductive structures, separately or in combination, seems rewarding in elucidating the process. *Helianthus annuus* L. may provide useful informations in this regard. The present work is therefore, undertaken with a view to understanding the source-sink relationship in relation to foliar senescence and yield of *Helianthus annuus,* which is also an important oil yielding plant.

Materials and Methods

Surface sterilized and water-soaked seeds of *Helianthus annuus* were sown in parallel lines in the garden, previously prepared with rotted farm-yard manure in the month of July. One week after emergence, plants in each row were thinned leaving a space of 60 cm in between the plants, watering was done at regular intervals.

Eighty flowers of similar age group (having two different sizes) were selected. Four different sets of flowers were maintained. For each set, 20 flowers were taken. Among the 40 small sized flowers, a separate set of 20 flowers maintained, where only one side shoot with an apical capitulum was allowed to grow from the axil of 3rd leaf. In case of hot water having a desired temperature (± 65°C) for a definite period (10 minutes) at anthesis stage.

For the determination of foliar senescence % of degradation of chlorophyll levels in 1st, 2nd and 3rd leaves (counted from top) was observed at an interval of 15 days until almost yellowing of leaves of any one of the above sets. Seed weight were also measured.

Results and Discussion

In normal condition, the degradation of chlorophyll in all leaves (1st, 2nd and 3rd) on the peduncle of large capitulum was faster compared to leaves on small capitulum (Table 1). At the initial stage the level of chlorophyll in the 3rd leaf (lacking side shoot) on both the penduncles was lower, but at the later stages become higher compared to 1st leaf. The rate of chlorophyll degradation in the 3rd leaf was always greater compared to other leaf (1st and 2nd), when it subtended a side shoot. The ultimate pattern of chlorophyll level (prior to harvest stage) among the three leaves in such plant from increasing to decreasing order was : 2nd > 1st > 3rd. In hot water treated flowers, the pattern of degradation of chlorophyll among the leaves on the peduncle was always sequential (3rd > 2nd > 1st), which was quite different from other sets. Reduction in dry wt of seeds was achieved when the capitulum subtended a side shoot. No seed formation on hot-water treated flowers. In normal condition, the earlier senescence of all leaves (1st, 2nd and 3rd) on the peduncle of large capitulum may be due to its greater participation in seed filling (increased in seed wt) compared to the leaves having small capitulum. In both the above sets, 1st leaf senesced earlier compared to older 2nd and 3rd leaf as it is closest to the capitulum (deleterious effect of senescence signal of the apical flower), though the loss of chlorophyll in 3rd leaf was higher at the initial stage. The level of chlorophyll in the 3rd leaf was always lower when it subtended a side shoot favours the nutrient exhaustion theory of senescence (Biswas and Mandal 1987). Here seed weight was also reduced.

In hot-water treated flowers the pattern of degradation of chlorophyll among the leaves was always 3rd > 2nd > 1st due to ageing phenomena (as the seeds were absent), where nutrients seem to be recovered from such leaves and consequently redirected towards the stem.

Table 4 : Percent of Degradation of Chlorophyll Compared to Normal

Treatments	*Flower age (days)*			
	30 *70% blooming*	*45* *100% blooming*	*60* *harvesting*	*Seed wt.*
Control				
Flower wt (45 g)				
1st leaf	5%	25%	90%	35g.
2nd leaf	7	18	75	
3rd leaf	10	20	80	
Flower wt (40 g)				
1st leaf	5	22	80	31.2
2nd leaf	7	10	60	
3rd leaf	8	15	75	
Flower wt (45 g)				
1st leaf	5	22	75	30
2nd leaf	8	11	65	
3rd leaf*	10	25	75	
Hot–H_2O treatment				
1st leaf	5	10	40	....
2nd leaf	5	11	45	
3rd leaf	7	14	50	

*Emergence of lateral shoot.

4.5 Comparative Study of Monocarpic Senescence of a Monocot (*Commelina benghalensis* L.) and a Dicot (*Oxalis corniculata L.*) : Migration of Senescence Signal Vs. Nutrient Drainage

Abstract

Prior to harvest all the parameters (chlorophyll, protein, sugar, dry weight) relating to yield and senescence were higher in two deflorated plant species than defruited or control plants indicating the senescence pattern as control > defruited > deflorated. So, aerial (chasmogamous) flowers are more lethal than the underground fruits to induce better yield and whole plant senescence.

Introduction

Most of the dicots and monocots follow a pattern which favours the concept that migration of a 'senescence signal' from the reproductive sink to the leaves (Nooden, 1988) causes foliar senescence. Though a few dicots and monocots follow the pattern where nutrient withdrawal from the foliar organs causes monocarpic senescence of such plants (Gover *et. al*, 1985). According to Biswas and Mandal (1993) both the above hypotheses (senescence signal and nutrient drainage) might act in a superimposing manner and is very difficult to separate them in a strict sense. *Commelina benghalensis* and *Oxalis corniculata* may be the useful edible herbals for the study of both 'senescence signal' and 'nutrient drainage' hypotheses since cleistogamous flowers situated below the leaves mature into fruits and act as a strong sink. By contrast, aerial flowers do not mature into fruits and therefore may act only as a supply of senescence signal. The present study aims at separating the role of aerial flowers and underground fruits in relation to their combined effect (control plants) and also analysing the senescence pattern of leaves during source-sink manipulation so as to get a clear picture about the correlative aspects of whole plant senescence of such two wildly grown ethnobotanically important leafy vegetables. No attempt has yet been made to study the foliar senescence of weeds in relation to their reproductive development. Our laboratory is also pioneer in the field of research on correlative regulation of whole plant senescence.

Materials and Methods

Both the weeds prefer moist sandy soil and generally grows during the rainy season in the shady waste places. For easy procurement both the weeds are developed (*Commelina benghalensis* from seeds and *Oxalis corniculata* propagated vegetatively) in moist sandy beds during July. Watering was done as and when required. For each 3 sets of experiment, 20 plants were manipulated through the modification of source and sink capacities :

(*i*) The plants were deflorated (only the aerial flowers were pinched off at the age of 50 days to 105 days).

(*ii*) Defruited by digging the soil without causing injury to the root system till the fruit setting from the plant age of 60 to 110 days.

(*iii*) Non-excised plants served as control.

For the assessment of senescence and source-sink relationship, chlorophyll, protein, sugar level of leaves alongwith dry weight of plants were estimated at the age of 115 days. The chlorophyll was extracted from 10 mg randomized samples of leaves with chilled acetone (–4°C) and the values were estimated at 660nm in a spectrochem spectrophotometer according to Arnon (1949). After removing the chlorophyll the same samples were washed 3 times with trichloroacetic acid (18%) and the residue dissolved in 1 ml of 0.5 M NaOH at 85°C for 1 hr. After removing the tissue debris, the protein was estimated with the Folin-phenol reagent (Lowry *et. al.*, 1951). For the estimation of dry weight the plants were oven-dried at 80°C for 12 hr. Extraction of soluble sugar was done from the oven-dried and powdered randomized samples of leaves as collected for chlorophyll estimation. The plant material alongwith 5ml glass-distilled water was autoclaved (15 lbs pressure) for 15 minutes and then centrifuged at 10,000 g for 10 minutes. The supernatant was used for the estimation of soluble sugar with 0.2% anthrone reagent (McCready *et al*, 1950). Data were statistically analysed by taking the source of variances as days, replication and error. The CD (critical difference) values were calculated (Panse and Sukhatme, 1967) at the significance level $P = 0.05$.

Results and Discussion

The chlorophyll level (Table) of the leaves of deflorated plants were higher than those of defruited and control plants indicating the senescence order for both the species as control

> defruited > deflorated. The maximum deferment of leaf senescence in deflorated plants may possibly be due to the absence of chasmogamous flowers, which might supply the senescence signal. Noodén (1984) stated that senescence signal developed from the fruits, migrates downwards for the induction of leaf senescence. It is concluded that the effect of nutrient withdrawal is less deleterious than senescence signal for the induction of senescence in both the medicinal weeds.

The level of protein (Table) in the leaves of deflorated plants increased compared to those of defruited and control plants may be due to non withdrawal of nutrients.

The level of sugar (Table) in the leaves of control plants increased compared to deflorated and defruited which support the direct correlation between sugar level and senescence.

Highest increase in aerial plant dry weight was found when the plants were deflorated. This findings indirectly favour the predominant role of aerial flowers to induce yield and senescence.

Table 5 : The Levels of Chlorophyll, Protein, Sugar and Dry Weight of Plants at the Plant Age of 115 Days (Prior to Harvest)

Treatments	*Chlorophyll mg/g FW^{-1}*	*Protein mg/g FW^{-1}*	*Sugar mg/g DW^{-1}*	*Dry weight g/$plant^{-1}$*
Control				
Commelina sp.	0.61	21.1	269	25.2
Oxalis sp.	0.65	22.2	268	20.1
Defruited				
Commelina sp.	0.81	39.1	265	26.1
Oxalis sp.	0.84	40.2	261	21.2
Deflorated				
Commelina sp.	0.85	40.3	261	28.2
Oxalis sp.	0.95	41.5	259	22.5
CD at 5%	0.14	4.12	12.2	0.65

References

Crafts-Brandner S.J. 1992, Phosphorus nutrition influence on leaf senescence in soybean. Plant Physiol. 98:1128-1132.

Arnon DI 1949, Copper enzymes in isolated chloroplasts. Polyphenol Oxidase in *Beta vulgaris*. Plant Physiol 241–15.

Niwa, T.; Doi, U.; Kato, Y. and Osawa, T. (2001). Antoxidant properties of phenolic antioxidants isolated from corn steep liquor. J. Agric Food Chem, 49, 177–182.

Tiwari, A.K. (2001). Imbalance in antioxidant defence and human disease. Multiple approach of natural antioxidants therapy. Curr Sci; 81(9), 1179–1187.

Ghosh, A. (2005). How one can survive for a long time in the earth. Ageing and Society. 15(3–4), 75–81.

Arnon, D.I. Copper enzymes in isolated chloroplasts, Polyphenol oxidase in *Beta vulgaris. Plant Physiol.*, 1949, 24, 1–15.

Biswas, A.K. and Mandal, S.K. Whole plant senescence in *Pennisetum typhoides* : implication of source-sink relationship. *J. Plant Physiol.*, 1987, 127, 371–377.

Ghosh, A.K. Mechanism of monocarpic senescence of *Trichosanthes dioica, Pak. J. Sci. Ind. Res.*, 2002, 45, 212.

Ghosh, A.K. and Biswas, A.K. Source-sink relationship during monocarpic senescence of *Raphanus sativus. Agri. Biol. Res.*, 1991, 7, 132–138.

Ghosh, A.K. and Biswas, A.K. Regulation of correlative senescence in *Arachis hypogaea* L. by source-sink alteration through physical and hormonal means. *J. Agron. Crop Sci.*, 1995, 175, 195–202

Lowry, O.H., Rosebrough, N.J., Farr, A.L. and Randall, R.J. Protein measurement with the folin phenol reagent. *J. Biol Chem.*, 1951, 193, 265–275.

McCready, R.M., Guggloz, J., Silviera, V. and Owens, H.S. Determination of starch and amylase in vegetables, *Ann. Chem.*, 1950, 22, 1156–1158.

Nooden, L.D. Senescence in the whole plant, In : *Senescence in Plant*, (ed.) K.V. Thiman, CRC Press, Boca Raton, Florida, 1980. pp. 219–258.

Nooden, L.D. Integration of soybean pod development and monocarpie senescence. *Physiol Plantarum*, 1984, 62, 273–284

Panse, V.G. and Sukhatme, P.T. *Statistical Methods for Agricultural Workers.* 2nd ed. ICAR, New Delhi, 1967.

Biswas A.K., Chaudhuri M.A. 1980. Mechanism of monocarpic senescence in rice. Plant Physiol **65** : 340–345.

Biswas A.K., Ghosh A.K. 1989. Monocarpic senescence in relation to yield of *Sesamum indicum during* source-sink alteration. J. Agron Crop Sci **162** : 342–346.

Biswas A.K., Mandal S.K. 1987. Whole plant senescence in *Pennisetum typhoides* : Implication of source-sink relationship. J Plant Physiol **127**: 371–377.

Chouduri M.A. Mandal W.A. 1988. Mechanism of monocarpic senescence in rice. Indian Rev Life Sci **8** : 3–28.

Nooden L.D. 1984. Integration of soybean pod development and monocarpic senescence. Physiol Plant **62** : 273–284.

Whitehead CS, Halevy A.H. 1989. Ethylene sensitivity : The role of short–chair saturated fatty acids in pollination–induced senescence of *Patunia hybrida* flowers. Plant Growth Regulation **8** : 41–54.

Arnon D.I. (1949). Copper enzymes in isolated chloroplasts. Polyphenol oxidase in *Beta vulgaris. Plant Physiol* **24** : 1–15.

Biswas A.K. and Mandal S.K. (1993). Senescence of flag leaf and glumes in rice : Role of grains during source-sink modification by physical and chemical means. *J. Agron. Crop Sci.* **171 :** 13–19.

Grover A., Koundal K.R. and Sinha S.K. (1985). Senescence of attached leaves : Regulation by developing pods. *Physiol plant.* **63 :** 87–92.

Lowry O.H., Rosebrough N.J., Farr A.I. and Randall R.I. (1951). Protein measurement with the folin phenol reagent. *J. Biol Chem.* **193 :** 265–275.

Mc Cready R.M., Guggloz J., Silviera V. and Owens H.S. (1950). Determination of starch and amylase in vegetables. *Ann Chem.* **22 :** 1156–1158.

Noodén L.D. (1984) Intetration of soybean pod development and monocarpic senescence. *Physiol Plant.* **62 :** 273–284.

Noodén L.D. (1988). Whole plant senescence. In senescence and aging in plants. L.D. Noodén and A.C. Leopold eds. Academic Press, San-Diego. pp. 391–439.

Panse V.G. and Sukhatme P.T. (1967). Statistical methods for agricultural workers, 2nd edn. ICAR, New-Delhi, pp. 150–157.

5

Epilogue

UTILIZATION OF VEILED POTENTIAL NATURAL RESOURCES FOR MANKIND

Exploration of indigenous process for developing excellent natural lustrous showy red 'Banak clay dye' obtained from underground soil (1–2.5 m depth in the crop fields) which is used in colouring tiles, dolls, earthen pitchers, cooking pots, bricks and walls etc.

My new findings for achieving desire qualities of honey for particular ailment from detached desirable apiphilic plant part in off season is worth emulating.

Tailoring of haulms serve as a natural remedy against Late blight of potato and as biofertilizer.

A domestic nutritious self-made baby food called 'Sneha' is prepared by me from roasted wheat and green-gram in 4:1 ratio. It is now widely popular among the self-supporting women group. Besides poor mans' drink is made from freshly collected dechlorophyllated pan (*Piper betle*) leaves alongwith the proportionate ingredients like citric acid, cumin, ginger, pepper, rock salt and sugar.

Application of organic manure to crops has been found useful to control hazardous effect of chemical manure. Biofertilizers is now being used to enhance plant growth, taste and reduce disease incidence in various crops. Water hyacinth (*Eichhornia crassipes*) leaves extract is spread on brinjal, potato, tomato crops to obtain luxuriant growth.

Proper utilization of various sewage by inoculation of *Eichhornia crassipes* and *Azolla pinnata* and thereby production of biofertilizer through abatement of sewage pollution. Exploration of naturally available suitable sand-binding plants in the coastal area.

Hope that my ample remarkable findings will prove useful in the daily life of common people, and this diversified use of natural resource is essential for future survival. Besides knowledge mapping and gathering can provide valuable leads for developing contemporary products.

Glossary of Ecological Terms

1. **Afforestation :** It is a process in which a large scale tree planting is carried out in open land and barren hills.
2. **Biodegradable :** Certain organic or inorganic substances could be easily destroyed by micro-organisms through decomposition process.
3. **Biomass :** Total weight of all the organisms in a particular habitat.
4. **Biosphere :** The envelope containing all the living things on earth.
5. **BOD :** Biological O_2 demand. It is the amount of O_2 required by micro-organisms in the water to carry out the decomposition process aerobically used as a measure in determining the contamination status of the water.
6. **Biotic Stability :** Ability of the population to live in an equilibrium or stable condition with an environment even after disturbance.
7. **Calorimeter :** An instrument used to measure the amount of energy in a given substance.
8. **Canopy :** The upper portion of the tree viewed from the sky.
9. **Climax Vegetation :** The last stage but the most stable condition within an ecological succession of communities.
10. **Decomposers :** Micro-organisms which lead the life by breaking down the dead organic matters in order to obtain energy.

11. **Deforestation** : The process by which trees are being out.
12. **Desertification** : Creation of desert like situation artificially by human activity.
13. **Ecology** : The study of the relationship between organisms and their environment.
14. **Ecosystem** : A system in ecology where organisms interact with each other for their survival.
15. **Ecotone** : Zone of transition between 2 vegetational regions.
16. **Energy Crops** : Crops grown to obtain energy from them (*e.g.* sugarcane provides ethanol, a potential substitute for conventional fuel such as petrol).
17. **Energy Flow** : Trapping of solar energy by photosynthetic organisms and its trasformation into chemical energy and passes through various trophic levels.
18. **Environment** : Sum of all external forces or influences that affect an organism.
19. **Euphotic Zone** : A layer of the water body especially the surface where organisms can photosynthesize with the help of light.
20. **Eutrophication** : The process occurring when the level of nutrients (organic) in a body of water increases markedly leading to an increase in the number of aquatic organisms.
21. **Field-Water Capacity** : The maximum amount of capillary water that a particular soil is able to hold.
22. **Forestry** : Science which concentrate on how to produce forest goods.
23. **Gene Pool** : Collection of genetically similar or dissimilar organisms.
24. **Grazing Food Chain** : The food chain in which animals eat the primary producers.

25. **Green House Effect :** Ability of the atmosphere to act like a green house where heat is retained by the glass wall. In atmosphere certain gasses trap and retain the heat.

26. **Green Manure :** Nutrients produced from the green plants to use as fertilizers.

27. **Gross Primary Production :** The rate at which solar energy is converted into chemical energy per unit of earth surface per unit time.

28. **Habitat :** Natural environment of plant or animal.

29. **Humus :** Organic matters formed in the forest soil due to decomposition of fallen leaves.

30. **Hydrosere :** Succession which starts from the aquatic system.

31. **Ice Cap Analysis :** Measurement of CO_2 concentration in the ancient snow on ice caps of glaciers.

32. **Laterite :** Reddish infertile tropical soil because of intense leaching out of silica; only Fe and Al rich clay is left, remains fertile only when a considerable amount organic matter is added continuously.

33. **Lentic Water :** Standing water bodies such as water of ponds or pool etc.

34. **Lianes :** Twining vines with woody stems.

35. **Litter :** A layer of undecomposed plant parts on the surface of the ground.

36. **Lotic Water :** Running water bodies of river etc.

37. **Monocroping :** Practice of cultivating only one kind of crop plant for many seasons.

38. **Mono Culture :** Practice of growing one kind of tree for commercial purposes.

39. **Mulching :** Practice of covering surface soil for maize stalks, cotton stalks, tobacco stalks, potato tops etc.

40. **Natality :** Death rate of a population.

41. **Net Primary Productivity :** The gross primary production minus, the amount of chemical energy used in respiration.

42. **Nuclear Waste :** Used radioactive substances of nuclear power stations.

43. **Oil Slick :** The floating layer of oil on the surface of water bodies.

44. **Ozone :** The thin layer which forms as a part of the upper atmosphere which filters out ultra-violet light from the sun.

45. **Polyploidy :** A process in which chromosome number doubles due to failed meiosis which results in the formation of new species.

46. **Population :** Group of related individuals capable of inter breeding.

47. **Primary Succession :** A succession beginning with bare or uninhabited area.

48. **Productivity :** Rate of dry-matter production by photosynthesis in an ecosystem.

49. **Pugmark :** Foot print of wild animals. During survey by measuring the pugmark the population of tiger, lion etc can be detected.

50. **Pyrolysis :** Subjecting biomass to 400°C to extract energy from it.

51. **Quadrat :** A frame of any shape, which when placed over vegetation defines a unit sample area within which the plants may be counted.

52. **Radiation :** Stream of particles or rays which are emitted by certain naturally occurring elements like U^{235}, radium 226 etc.

53. **Remote Sensing :** Technique of taking photograph of landscape from the airborne or space borne platform.

54. **Savanna :** A tropical grassland consisting of tall, coarse grasses and scattered small trees.

55. **Secondary Succession** : A succession that begins with the disturbed remains of a previous vegetation.

56. **Soil Profile :** The structure and composition of a soil as seen in the side of a pit, trench etc.; made up of layers or horizons produced by leaching and deposition.

57. **Steady State :** State in which the inflow of energy and materials in an ecosystem is just sufficient to maintain biomass at a relatively constant level.

Glossary of Medical Terms

Abscess	A localized collection of pus in any part of the body. The result of disintegration of displacement of tissue.
Abortifacient	Anything used to cause or induce an abortion.
Ague	A popular name for malarial fever.
Alexeteric	Protective against infection, venom and poison.
Alexephermic	Antidotal.
Alternative	A drug which corrects disorder process of nutrition and restores the normal function of an organ or of the system.
Amenorrhoea	Suppression of menses not due to natural causes.
Anaemia	Condition in which there is a reduction in the number of circulating red blood per cu. mm, the amount of haemoglobin per 100 ml of blood.
Anodyne	A drug that relieves pains : an analgesic.
Anthelmintic	An agent that destroys parasitic intestinal worms.
Antithydrotic	A drug which checks sweating.
Antiperiodic	A drug which controls periodic attacks of disease; an anti-malarial drug.

Antispasmidic	A drug which prevents or cures colic, convulsions or spasmodic disorders.
Antipyretic	Reducing fever. An agent that reduces fever.
Antidote	A substance that neutralizes poisons or their effect.
Antisyphilitic	Curative or relieves syphilis.
Antiseptic	An agent capable of producing antiseposis.
Anticholinergic	Impending the impulses of cholinergic neurotransmitters. An agent that blocks parasympathetic nerve impulses.
Anthrax	Acute, infectious disease caused by *Bacillus anthracis*, usually attacking cattle, sheep, horses and goats. Man contracts it from contact with animal hairs, hides or waste.
Aperient	A laxative or mild purgative.
Aphrodisiac	A drug which promotes sexual desire.
Apoplexy	Sudden loss of consciousness followed by paralysis caused by hemorrhage in the brain.
Aromatic	A drug having an agreeable odor.
Ascarides	A collection of fluid in the abdomen, abdominal dropsy.
Asthma	A disease of the bronchial tubes causing recurrent attacks of breathlessness and coughing.
Astringent	To bind fast, drawing together, constricting, binding. An agent that has a constricting or binding effect; *i.e.* one that checks hemorrhage or secretions by coagulation of proteins on a cell surface.

Benzaldehyde	A pharmaceutical flavouring agent derived from oil of better almond.
Billiousness	A symptom of a disordered condition of the liver causing constipation, headache, loss of appetite and vomiting of bile.
Black water fever	Billious remittent fever, a complication of malaria.
Belennorrhoea	Excessive mucous discharge, particularly from the urethra or vaginal gonorrhoea.
Blister	An accumulation of the fluid under the upper layer of the skin; a substance applied to the skin for raising a blister.
Boil	An infectious festering sore which ultimately may develop into an ulcer.
Bright's disease	An acute or chronic disease of kidneys.
Bronchitis	An inflammation of mucous membrane of the bronchial tubes or air passage; feverish cold with cough and sore chest.
Bruises	An injury with diffuse effusion into sub-cutaneous tissue and in which skin is discoloured but not broken.
Cardiac	Pertaining to heart.
Cardiotonic	Increasing tonicity of the heart. Various drugs, including digitalis, are cardiotonic.
Carminative	A drug which relieves flatulence or the feeling of over-fulness of the stomach.
Catarrh	Term formerly applied to inflammation of mucous membranes, especially of head and throat.
Cathartic	An active purgative producing bowel movements.
Cerebral	Pertaining to cerebrum, the brain.

Cholangogue	An agent that increases the flow of bile into the intestine.
Chorea	A nervous condition marked by involuntary muscular twitching of the limbs or facial muscles.
Colic	Spasm in any hollow or tubular soft organ accompanied by pain.
Cutaneous	Pertaining to skin.
Cystitis	Inflammation of bladder.
Dandruff	Normal exfoliation of the epidermis of the scalp in the form of dry white scales.
Demulcent	Stroking softly. An agent that will smooth the part of soften the skin to which applied.
Depressant	An agent that reduces functional activity.
Delirium	A state of mental confusion and excitement characterized by disorientation.
Depurative	Having cleaning properties; removing waste material from the body. Removal of waste material.
Deodorant	Perfumoral. An agent that masks or absorbs foul odours.
Diaphoretic	An agent that increase perspiration, such as camphor, opium or pilocarpine. Heat may also be included as such an agent. An agent that induces copious secretion of sweat.
Diarrhoea	Frequent passage of unformed watery bowel movement. It is a frequent symptom of gastrointestinal disturbance.
Diathesis	Constitutional predisposition to a certain disease, condition or group of diseases. Can be allergic, hemorrhagic or rheumatic disease.

Diabetes	A general term for diseases characterized by excessive urination. Usually refers to Diabetes mellitus.
Dropsy	Disease causing a watery fluid to collect in some cavity of the body.
Diuretic	An agent that increases the secretion of urine.
Dyspepsia	Imperfect or painful digestion. Not a disease in itself but symptomatic of other diseases or disorders, indigestion.
Dysentery	An infectious disease, characterized by acute diarrhoea accompanied by gripping pains, the stools being chiefly of blood and mucous.
Dysuria	Painful and difficult urination.
Dysmenorrhoea	Pain in association with menstruation. One of the most frequent gynecologic disorders.
Eczema	Itching skin disease.
Elephantiasis	A disease of the skin and subcutaneous tissues causing hypertrophy of the affected parts. It may attack any part of the body but chiefly attacks the legs.
Emetic	An agent that produces vomiting.
Emollient	An agent that will soften and soothe the part when applied locally.
Emmenagogue	A substance that promotes or assists the flow of menstrual fluid.
Epilepsy	Nervous disease causing a person to fall unconscious (often with violent involuntary movement).
Expectorant	An agent that facilitates the removal of the secretion of the bronchopulmonary mucous

	membranes. Classified as sedative or stimulating.
Febrifuge	An agent or drug used for reducing fever.
Febrile	Pertaining to fever, feverish.
Flatulence	Excessive gas in the stomach and intestines.
Freckles	Coloured spots, generally yellowish or brown, on the exposed parts on the skin.
Fructose	Levulose, fruit sugar.
Galactagogue	An agent that promotes the secretion and flow of milk; lactagogue.
Glect	A mucous discharge from the urethra in chronic gonorrhoea.
Gonorrhoea	A specific contagious, catarrhal inflammation of the genital mucous membranes of either sex.
Gravel	The development in the kidneys and urinary tract of tiny stone-like collection of uric acid, calcium oxalate or phosphates.
Granulation	Formation of granules or slate or condition of being granular.
Griping	A sharp policy pain in the bowels due to presence of some irritating substance.
Haematuria	Passing of blood in the urine.
Haemorrhage	Bleeding, especially profuse, from any part of the body.
Haemorrhoids	Piles; a diseased condition of the blood vessels causing painful swellings in the region of the anus.
Hemicrania	Headache on only one side of the head; migraine.
Hepatitis	Inflammation of the liver.

Herpes	Creeping skin diseases.
Hernia	The protrusion or projection of an organ or a part of an organ through the wall of the cavity that normally contains it.
Hiccough	Spasmodic periodic closure of the glottis following spasmodic lowering the diaphragm, causing a short sharp, inspiratory cough.
Hydrophobia	Morbid fear of water. Common name of rabies resulting from bite of rabid animal.
Hysteria	A disease in which the patient who is physically healthy, suffers from imaginary diseases and has lost control over acts and feelings.
Hypnotic	Pertaining to sleep or hypnosis. An agent that induces sleep or that dulls the senses, such as chloral hydrate.
Induration	Area of hardened tissues.
Insomnia	An excessive amount of fibrin in the blood.
Intermittent	Suspending activity and intervals. Coming and going.
Ipacacauanha	It is a plant grown in Brazil. The dried root of this plant is known as Ipacacauanha. It is the source of emetine q.v.
Itch	An infectious disease of skin without specific lesions and marked by excessive itching.
Jaundice	A disease condition of the liver in which there is yellowish colouring of the tissues and urine with bile.
Laryngitis	Inflammation of larynx.

Leprosy	A chronic wasting disease caused by a germ which generally, results in mutilations and deformities.
Leucoderma	A skin disease marked by skin losing its pigment wholly or partially.
Leucorrhoea	A vaginal discharge of a white fluid containing mucous or pus cells.
Lithiasis	The formation of calculi or stone in any part of the body.
Lithotriptic	A drug having the property of crushing a calculus in or stone present in the urinary system.
Lithositic	Having the property of crushing a calculus in the bladder or urethra.
Lumbago	Rheumatism of the small of the back causing acute pain and stiffness.
Mania	Mental disorder characterized by excessive excitement.
Melancholia	A disorder of the mind marked by depression of spirits, mental sluggishness and apathy to ones surroundings.
Menorrhagia	Abnormally excessive menstruation.
Micturition	Urination.
Migraine	A nervous disorder marked by periodic attacks of headache; hemicrania.
Mucilaginous	Resembling mucilage, slimy; sticky.
Mumps	An infectious disease marked by inflammation of glands near the ear.
Mydriatic	A drug which dilates the pupil
Narcotic	A drug which induces deep sleep or insensibility to pain.

Nausea	A feeling of sickness; inclination to vomit.
Nephritis	Inflammation of the kidneys.
Neuralgia	Severe sharp pain along the course of nerves.
Opthalmia	Inflammation of the nerves; conjunctivitis.
Otitis	Inflammation of the ear.
Otorrhoea	A purulent discharge from the ear.
Palsy	Temporary or permanent loss of sensation or loss of ability to move or to control movement.
Paralysis	Loss of motion in any fraction of any part of the body.
Paroxysms	A sudden, periodic attack or recurrence of symptoms of a disease. Sudden spasm or convulsion of any kind. Sudden emotional state, as of fear, grief or joy.
Pectoral	Pertaining to the chest; cough remedy; expectorant.
Photophobia	Unusual intolerance of light.
Phithisis	Affected with pulmonary tuberculosis.
Piles	An inflammed condition of veins in the rectal region; haemorrhoids.
Pleurisy	Inflammation of the membrane enclosing the lungs.
Pneumonia	Inflammation of the lungs.
Polyploidy	Condition in which the chromosome number is two or more times the normal haploid number found in gamets.
Poultice	A hot, moist mass of linseed, mustard or soap and oil between two pieces of muslin applied to the skin to relieve conjection or

	pain, to stimulate absorption of inflammatory products, and to act as a counter irritant.
Prolapse	A falling down of an organ from its normal position, especially its appearance at an opening.
Pruritus	Severe itching. May be a symptom of a disease process such as allergic response or be due to emotional factors.
Pulmonary	Pertaining to lings.
Pungent	Sharp smell or taste.
Pyorrhoea	A purulent discharge from the gums.
Pyrosis	A burning sensation in the epigastric and sternal region with raising of acid liquid from stomach.
Rectum	Lower part of large intestine.
Refrigerant	An agent which relieves feverishness or produces a feeling of coolness.
Refringent	Refractive.
Rheumatism	A term used for pains in the muscles, joints and certain tissues; the disease takes various forms.
Resolvent	Promoting disappearance of inflammation.
Rubefacient	A mild counter-irritant; a drug that causes tingling reddening of the skin.
Sciatica	A neuralgic pain at the back of the thigh caused by the inflammation of the sciatica nerve.
Scorbutic	Suffering from scurvy.
Scrofula	A disease chiefly of the young, marked by want of resisting power making the patient

	susceptible to tuberculosis especially of the glands, bones and joints, eczematous eruption, ulceration, glandular swelling, etc.
Sedative	A drug which has a calming or quieting effect on the patient and which reduces nervous excitement.
Sialagogue	A drug which promotes the secretion of saliva.
Soporific	A drug that induces sleep.
Spasmophile	A tendency to tetany and convulsion; almost always association with rickets.
Spasmodic	A convulsion. Concerning spasms.
Stomatitis	Inflammation of the mucous membrane of the mouth.
Stomachic	A drug which improves digestion and appetite.
Strangury	Painful and drop by drop discharge of urine.
Styptic	An agent which checks bleeding.
Sudroific	An agent that promotes perspiration; a diaphoretic.
Suppuration	The process of pus formation.
Syphilis	A serious chronic venereal disease.
Taenia	Tapeworms.
Tetanus	An infectious disease, marked by painful contractions in the muscles.
Tinea	A group of parasitic skin diseases, ringworm.
Tonsillitis	Inflammation of tonsil.
Trachoma	A contagious granular inflammation of the conjective.

Tuberculosis	A disease caused by bacillus; it may affect any part of organ of the body.
Ulcer	An open sore on the skin or on any mucous membrane.
Vermifuge	A drug which expels intestinal worms.
Vertego	Dizziness; giddiness.
Vesicant	A drug or agent that produces blisters.
Vulnerary	A drug which promotes healing of wounds.
Wart	A hypertrophy or growth on the skin.
Whooping cough	An acute infectious disease marked by recurring peculiar spasmodic attacks of coughing, each attack ending with a deep noisy intake of breath.

Plant Index

T

V

W

Z